P9-DTM-417

DATE DUE

DEMCO 38-296

BIOCULTURAL DIMENSIONS OF CHRONIC PAIN

SUNY Series in Medical Anthropology
Setha Low, editor

BIOCULTURAL DIMENSIONS OF CHRONIC PAIN

Implications for Treatment of Multi-Ethnic Populations

Maryann S. Bates

STATE UNIVERSITY OF NEW YORK PRESS

Riverside Community College
Library
4800 Magnolia Avenue
Riverside, CA 92506

RB 127 .B374 1996

Bates, Maryann S., 1942-

Biocultural dimensions of
 chronic pain

Published by
State University of New York Press, Albany

© 1996 State University of New York

All rights reserved

Printed in the United States of America

No part of this book may be used or reproduced
in any manner whatsoever without written permission.
No part of this book may be stored in a retrieval system
or transmitted in any form or by any means including
electronic, electrostatic, magnetic tape, mechanical,
photocopying, recording, or otherwise without the
prior permission in writing of the publisher.

For information, address State University of New York
Press, State University Plaza, Albany, N.Y., 12246

Production by Cathleen Collins
Marketing by Theresa Abad Swierzowski

Library of Congress Cataloging-in-Publication Data

Bates, Maryann S., 1942–1995
    Biocultural dimensions of chronic pain : implications for
 treatment of multi-ethnic populations / Maryann S. Bates.
       p.   cm. — (SUNY series in medical anthropology)
    Includes bibliographical references and index.
    ISBN 0–7914–2735–8 (hardcover). — ISBN 0–7914–2736–6
 (pbk.)
       1. Chronic pain—Cross-cultural studies. I. Title. II. Series.
    [DNLM: 1. Pain—ethnology.   2. Pain—psychology.   3. Chronic
 Disease.   4. Attitude to Health—ethnology.   5. Cross-Cultural
 Comparison.   WL 704 B329b 1996]
    RB 127.B374   1996
    616'.0472'01—dc20
    DNLM/DLC
    For Library of Congress   95–15487
                                                                          CIP

10 9 8 7 6 5 4 3 2 1

*In Memory of the Best Physician
I Have Ever Known*

Ricardo Mendez Bryan, M.D.

This book is dedicated to my husband,
Murray Bates,
whose constant support, love and critical reviews
made this book possible;

and to my parents, Virginia and Frank Snow,
who, by example, taught me the value of hard work,
determination, and perseverance, thus giving me the
skills that enabled me to reach this goal.

CONTENTS

TABLES

FIGURES

INTRODUCTION

For the chronic pain sufferer, days are filled with endless pain that no one else can understand, and nights are even longer due to insomnia and pain that seems to worsen in the darkness. Often no one in the sufferer's family or social circle understands the pain or why the pain sufferer cannot get well. Months or years of biomedical evaluations and treatments and often treatments by alternative health-care providers have left the chronic pain sufferer emotionally, physically, and financially drained. The world of the chronic pain sufferer is a lonely one. Even for those who somehow come to terms with chronic intractable pain and find ways to function in their social and work worlds, pain is a constant companion, a part of one's life that friends, family, and colleagues do not wish to hear about and do not fully comprehend.

Pain is essential to human survival and is a condition known to all cultural groups. However, some people suffer with pain which is intractable, and which no longer serves as a signal in detecting potential or actual damage, and that is no longer beneficial to the sufferer or those who provide him or her with care in terms of diagnosing and treating an injury or illness. Such people suffer from chronic pain, which is now recognized as a serious health and economic problem. The estimated annual cost of chronic pain in the United States alone, in health care, drugs, disability compensation, lost wages, etc., is between fifty and ninety billion dollars (Lipton 1990:xxxi; Morris 1991:19). It is estimated that at least fifty and perhaps as many as ninety million people in just the United States suffer with chronic pain (Turk, Meichenbaum, and Genest 1983; Bonica 1985; Holzman and Turk 1986; Morris 1991). Chapter 1 provides a discussion of these "pain patients" (as they are characterized in the literature) and also presents two case studies of chronic pain sufferers whom I have worked with in the two studies described in this book. These cases contradict the myth in the chronic pain literature that all chronic pain sufferers are much alike and all have a similar chronic pain "career"[1] (Kotarba 1983; Aronoff 1985). Beginning in chapter 1 and throughout this book, I will demonstrate considerable diversity among the chronic pain sufferers who participated in the two studies described here.

Over the past twenty-five years there has been increased international research on chronic pain, and over 1,200 chronic pain treatment centers have emerged in the United States alone (Holzman and Turk 1986). An overview of current chronic pain treatment approaches is provided in chapter 2. Despite the high incidence and costs and the rapid increase in treatment facilities, effective treatments or cures for chronic pain remain elusive. Yet this book about the experiences of several hundred chronic pain sufferers is not necessarily pessimistic. As many of the case studies to be presented here demonstrate, despite biomedicine's failure to totally alleviate chronic pain in many such patients, many pain sufferers find ways to adapt their behaviors and attitudes that allow them to lead happy and fulfilled lives despite continued pain.

Theories of human pain perception have undergone radical changes over the last three decades. Previously, pain was conceptualized by the biomedical community as a strictly sensory experience occurring in response to potential or actual body damage; pain for which no such damage or pathology could be found was assumed to be of psychological origin (Bonica 1985:xxiii). This view is an extension of the traditional biomedical paradigm based on a mind-body dualism in which each particular medical problem or symptom is viewed as originating either in the body or in the mind.

In 1965, Melzack and Wall proposed a dramatically different model, the *gate-control theory*, of human pain perception. This revolutionary theory, to be described in detail in chapter 2, proposed that mental and physical processes interact in systematic ways in human pain perception. This theoretical perspective on human pain stimulated a great deal of discussion and many new research approaches. However, despite an increase in pain research during the past two decades, there is still much to be

---

1. The term chronic pain "career" is an indication of the judgmental and stereotypical attitude in the literature toward most chronic pain patients who are assumed to focus their attention almost exclusively on their pain and to have lives which revolve around the pain. In contrast to much of the literature (Aronoff 1985; Kotarba 1983), my research indicates many such patients have found ways to adjust attitudes and behaviors in order to lead what they define as happy and productive lives and have been able to continue to have meaningful social and/or work lives despite having the pain.

learned about the interaction of physiological, psychological, cognitive, sociocultural, and behavioral components in the human pain experience.

The two multidisciplinary studies described in this book use a biocultural approach from medical anthropology (Armelagos et al. 1978; Armelagos et al. 1992) as well as methods and theories from the field of chronic pain studies (algology) and from psychology, sociology and political economy. The studies were designed to determine the role of ethnic identity and cultural background in variations in the chronic pain experience and to develop a more thorough understanding of the interactions of biology and culture in the pain experience. The research also sought to determine social, psychological, and biological factors affecting the chronic pain experience and to delineate the elements in the complex physical, psychosocial, cultural, political, economic, and health-care environments which affect the experiences of chronic pain sufferers. The research was designed with an applied orientation and sought to provide insights that would contribute to the development of well-integrated, effective, and culturally appropriate multidisciplinary treatment and rehabilitation programs to assist multiethnic chronic pain populations.

Through individual case studies and presentation of qualitative and quantitive data analyses, this book contradicts the picture painted in much of the chronic pain literature, which often portrays chronic pain sufferers as devious and in some way gaining, emotionally and/or financially, from retaining their pain (Aronoff 1985:472). It will be demonstrated that by using cultural, psychosocial, and other resources, substantial numbers of chronic pain sufferers gradually find ways to adapt to their pain and lead meaningful, worthwhile, and productive lives. This book is written from the patients' perspectives and with great admiration for these people who live daily with chronic pain, yet somehow manage to fulfill social and work responsibilities to their families, employers, and communities.

Chapters 3, 4, and 5 present the results of a quantitative and qualitative study of the chronic pain experiences of 372 patients in six ethnic groups who were under treatment at an outpatient multidisciplinary pain-management center affiliated with a major university medical center in New England. The study was conducted during 1987 and 1988. In chapters 6 and 7, data are presented from a study conducted in Puerto Rico from 1990 to 1993 which investigated the chronic pain experiences of 100 island Puerto Ricans; comparisons between the Puerto Rican group and each of two groups from New England are also provided.

In chapter 8, the concluding chapter, a biocultural model for understanding the interactions of biology and culture in the human pain experience is detailed, the environmental context of the chronic pain sufferer is summarized, and the factors which influenced adaptation to chronic pain in these two studies are identified. Finally, suggestions for improving care, treatment, and rehabilitation of multiethnic chronic pain populations are offered.

In preparing this book and conducting the studies upon which it is based, I have benefited from the support of many individuals and agencies, whom I wish to acknowledge here. The two studies were funded by two National Science Foundation Grants (#BNS8705615 and #DBS-9120255); two Biomedical Research Support Grants (#SO7RR07149-16 and #SO7RR07149-19) from the Biomedical Research Support Grant Program, Division of Research Resources, National Institute of Health; a grant from Sigma Xi; several grants from the State University of New York at Binghamton; and a United University Professions New Faculty Development Award. My research leave to write this book was funded by the Naula M. Dreshcer Affirmative Action Program of New York State and the United University Professions. I am very grateful for the support of these institutions.

Most of all, I thank the patients of both centers for sharing their experiences with me and, in many cases, welcoming me into their homes. I am humbled by their willingness to share painful experiences as well as their triumphs with me. I will always be grateful for all that these study participants taught me.

I also want to extend my deepest appreciation and thanks to my dear colleagues and friends, Professors Lesley Rankin-Hill and Melba Sanchez, who were the Co-Principal Investigators on the Puerto Rican project. Dr. Rankin-Hill has spent endless hours discussing this research with me during its creation, implementation, and completion. Her ideas and knowledge of anthropology contributed to the development of the original biocultural model and to the overall success of the research and this book. I also especially want to thank Dr. W. Thomas Edwards and Dr. Ricardo Mendez Bryan for their cooperation and willingness to allow social science research at their institutions. Professors George J. Armelagos, Ralph H. Faulkingham, and Paula Stamps all deserve my gratitude and thanks for their immense help as I developed and researched the New England study. I also want to thank Professors Andy Anderson, Helen Ball, and Ann Magennis; Dr. Deborah Sellers; Yolanda Fernandez; Lydia Robles-Calderon; Anna Tuti Mendez; Anna Tutica Mendez; Mary Neilan; Debbie Hanna; Dominique Simon; Paulette Hackman; Steve Marion; and all of the physicians and staff of both centers for contributing to the successful completion and analysis of these projects.

Many thanks to my daughter, Jacqueline Gott, who helped prepare the final manuscript for publication and provided incredible support during some very difficult days. A special thanks also goes to Mary Cassandra (Timmy) Hill for her professional drawings of the models. I want to thank Dean Linda Biemer of the School of Education and Human Development at Binghamton University and Professor Joseph DeVitis of the Division of Human Development at Binghamton University for their support as I researched and wrote this book. I also wish to thank my editor at SUNY Press, Chris Worden, and the three anonymous reviewers whose helpful suggestions considerably improved the book.

Finally, I wish to express gratitude to Penguin Books, 27 Wrights Lane, London, England, for granting permission to use figures and quotes from the book *The Challenge of Pain* (1983, 1988) by R. Melzack and P. Wall.

CHAPTER 1

WORLDS OF PAIN

*Somewhere within us, say the pundits, there is a sensorium commune,
an undetermined site wherein the nature of pain is revealed. More
elusive than the Holy Grail for which medieval man sought widely and
in vain, the quest for the sensorium commune has preoccupied and frustrated [hu]man's thinking since time immemorial. To find it, and define
it, may resolve the probem of dealing with it; but, so far, biopsychosocial
research has only given new insights into the complexity of the quest.*
—Todd, *Pain: Historical Perspectives*

CHRONIC PAIN PATIENTS

"Pain patients," as chronic pain sufferers are generally referred to in the
medical and particularly in the psychological literature, often have been
defined as a relatively homogeneous group (Aronoff 1985:472; Kotarba
1983; Sternbach 1974, 1984; Lindsay and Wyckoff 1981; Fordyce 1976).
Aronoff's description of the stereotypical "chronic pain patient" provides
an excellent example. Director of the Boston Pain Center and one of the
leading American specialists in chronic pain, Aronoff states:

> These [pain] patients share many of the following characteristics:
> preoccupation with pain, strong and ambivalent dependency
> needs, feelings of isolation and loneliness, characterologic
> masochism (meeting other people's needs at their own expense),
> inability to take care of self-needs, passivity, lack of insight into
> patterns of self-defeating behavior, inability to deal appropri-
> ately with anger and hostility, and the use of pain as a symbolic
> means of communication. . . . Chronic pain can often represent
> conditioned psychosocioeconomic disorders in which personal
> gains may play an important role. (1985:472)

The widespread belief in a single, homogeneous "type" of chronic pain patient has led to homogeneous care and treatment programs which are ineffective for many patients. In many instances the failure of these programs is attributed to characteristics of the patients, who are assumed to be somewhat neurotic and in some way gaining from the pain (Aronoff, 1985). This is often a case of "blaming the victim." It is just as likely that the practitioners' inability to help these patients reflects a current lack of biomedical knowledge or the inflexibility of their programs, which cannot meet the needs of diverse populations that suffer from chronic pain.

Patients in the New England pain center and Puerto Rican populations to be presented in this book vary significantly in many ways: in cultural and psychological characteristics, in reported pain intensity, and in behavioral, cognitive, and psychological/emotional responses to pain. The diversity in these populations in coping strategies and day-to-day responses to the chronic pain experience is particularly clear in two case studies gathered from the Puerto Rican study. These case studies introduce us to the lived worlds of the chronic pain sufferer. (Fictitious names are used in the case studies to protect patient confidentiality.)

MEETING THE CHALLENGE OF PAIN: CASE STUDY NUMBER ONE

Manuel, a professional Puerto Rican with an advanced degree, is in his mid-fifties and was interviewed during 1992 and 1993 in Puerto Rico. He has had chronic pain associated with severe rheumatoid arthritis for more than fifteen years. The joints of his fingers are noticeably deformed, he walks with a limp, and he has severe arthritis in his fingers, hands, knees, hips, feet, toes, ankles, and spine. One of his hips has been replaced surgically. His physician believes Manuel should not be working at all, and that he urgently needs to have joint replacement surgery in several additional joints.

Manuel, however, refuses both of these prescriptions. He said his work keeps him going, and that he has no intention of stopping the work he loves or of having further surgery. Typical of other Puerto Rican men interviewed, Manuel believes his self-image, happiness, and "manhood" depend on his ability to work. When his arthritis became severe, one of his methods for adapting to his increasing pain and disability was to relocate his office to his home. Clients now travel to him, which reduces his travel and allows him to rest as needed. He said he considers himself fortunate, and he recognizes that if his employment involved manual labor he would have had to stop working long ago. However, with great determination and contrary to his physician's advice, he continues to work. During his busiest season, Manuel works many fifteen-or sixteen-hour days. He said he believes his work is the most important factor in coping and adapting to the pain.

On a visit to his office, it was clear Manuel had designed it to accommodate his arthritis. He had a sofa on which he could lie down as needed, special cushions on his desk chair, and a specially designed computer table and chair. Manuel's numerous topical remedies as well as his oral arthritis medications were handy and easily accessible.

He also is determined to continue his social activities. Married with three grown children, he loves to go to parties with his wife, and especially loves to dance. Despite one artificial hip and severe arthritis in his other hip, his knees, and his feet, Manuel continues to dance regularly. He said he recently had one of the worst days of his life in terms of pain intensity, although, he proudly said, he still went to an anniversary party and danced throughout the day. The pride and pleasure Manuel finds in dancing is understandable, as dancing is an integral part of the Puerto Rican social fabric (unless restricted by religion). In addition, being a good dancer is a highly regarded ability, especially for males.

Manuel told me, "You have to learn to live with the pain and forget about it. I always remember that there are others who are worse off than I am. I must keep my mind clear and continue to work and do the things I enjoy." In order to ensure the "clear mind" he values, Manuel deliberately takes only anti-inflammatory medications, and refuses opiates or other medications prescribed solely for pain.

Manuel said he has found ways to live with his pain and still work and enjoy his life. He clearly does not like to dwell on his condition, but was willing to discuss it as long as the focus was on how to cope with the pain effectively. He defines his status as "mainly healthy." Manuel exhibited a strong sense of having control over his life, and he clearly takes pride and satisfaction in his ability to adapt to the arthritis and to cope effectively. "I have a good life," he said.

In light of his determination to ignore his pain, it is not surprising that Manuel's score on the McGill Pain Questionnaire (MPQ), which is a standardized and widely used instrument for assessing pain quality and intensity levels, was very low and extremely low on its *affective* section of the questionnaire. Unlike the majority of Puerto Ricans of both genders who view expressiveness as appropriate, Manuel appears determined not to become emotional about his pain or to focus on it. He does admit, somewhat reluctantly, that the pain is occasionally tiring and troublesome, but for the most part he feels he can live with it as long as he can work and engage in pleasurable activities. When asked whether he was determined to overcome his pain, he responded, "I am not just determined to, I *do* overcome it."

DISABILITY, DESPAIR, AND CHRONIC PAIN: CASE STUDY NUMBER TWO

Our second Puerto Rican case study is Jesus, of middle-class background. He was in his forties when interviewed during 1990 and 1993. Although Manuel and Jesus share a similar cultural perspective on the importance of work to self-control, self-fulfillment, and sense of "maleness," Jesus has been unable to continue to work. As a result of Jesus's inability to continue working and the resulting loss of his self-esteem, his chronic pain experience differs significantly from Manuel's.

Like Manuel, Jesus also has an advanced degree, and prior to his pain problem he had a successful professional career. His position required both office work and frequent travel. Jesus reported that he felt in control of his life before developing severe postsurgical back problems following disk surgery approximately four years ago. (He also now has degenerative joint disease of the spine and arthritis in his knees.) However, since developing the chronic pain, he reported having lost all sense of control over his life.

Jesus wants desperately to return to some type of work; however, he is caught in the trap of the current disability system of the United States. He and his doctor believe he could work in an office for about four hours per day. Extensive travel is impossible. When Jesus and his doctor suggested to his disability benefits provider (which is the private insurance carrier for his old employer) that he work twenty hours per week for his old employer at the office (with the stipulation that he could not engage in travel), his old employer said he could only return to his position if he worked forty hours per week and did the same traveling he engaged in before the disability occurred. His disability compensation is tied to his old employer—thus his choice was to work forty hours per week and engage in extensive travel, or, if he wanted to work a twenty-hour week, give up his disability benefits through his old employer and try to find a new half-time position. Obviously, even if he could find such a position, it would not pay as well as the benefits which are based on his former forty-hours-per-week salary and he would permanently lose the current benefits, including his health insurance.

Jesus is the sole support of his wife and four children. He has significant financial responsibilities, with two children already in college and a third child only a year away from entering college. With disability compensation as the major source for financing his children's higher education, he sees no choice but to remain on disability—yet he feels worthless because he is not working.

As a result of his grave professional and financial concerns, Jesus reported to his center physician and at interviews that he is severely depressed and sees a psychologist regularly. He is a deeply unhappy man who sees little purpose in life and defines himself as unhealthy and disabled. He believes the pain has ruined his life. He said the pain and disability have taken away all control he once had over his life and that the accompanying inability to work has resulted in the loss of his manhood.

Resulting from his depression and despair, Jesus has attempted suicide more than once, as confirmed by his physician at the medical center, who was deeply worried about him. During several interviews, including two home visits, Jesus was greatly disturbed about his inability to work, to engage in sports with his teenage son, or to attend the boy's sports competitions. Despite having a very supportive wife, children he clearly adores, and a loving extended family, Jesus is unable to find any meaning and purpose in his life as long as he continues to have pain. He reported thinking constantly of his pain and disability.

Consistent with his view that only an outside person or force could influence his current circumstances, Jesus continues to seek the care and advice of a host of medical and psychological specialists. He has read about chronic pain treatment centers and wants to seek such services; however, no live-in treatment centers exist on the island. (Apparently the Medical Sciences Campus of the University of Puerto Rico had been developing an outpatient chronic pain clinic, which was not fully operational when we met with Jesus.) Upon the recommendation of his physician at the center, Jesus would seek care at an inpatient chronic pain treatment facility on the mainland, but his disability insurance company has refused to finance such treatment.[1] Very upset by the insurance company's decision, he said that unless he could attend a pain clinic or find a

---

1. The decision of the insurance company is obviously based on short-term economic considerations, as live-in chronic pain treatment centers are very expensive, and there is a perception, among "third-party payers, that pain program treatment for back pain is ineffective in attaining specific socioeconomic goals, such as cost effectiveness and return to work" (Tollison et al. 1989:1116). However, Tollison et al. found this perception to be inaccurate in their study of treatment outcome, which found that back-injured pain center patients participating in programs based on an industrial medicine model used fewer analgesics; required fewer hospitalizations for additional diagnoses, treatments, and surgery; and were more likely to return to work than a comparison group of patients denied comparable treatment (1115).

physician who could cure his pain and disability very soon, he would commit suicide.

Given his severe depression, Jesus's desire to return to some type of work should not be ignored, as Dworkin et al. (1986) found that activity is especially important in the treatment of depressed chronic pain patients. However, the disability system, as well as an inflexible former employer, contribute to the problems Jesus faces. Even for professionals such as Jesus, with private disability insurance rather than workers' compensation, the current system offers little help to those who want to return to work but need a restructured work environment or flexible work schedule to accommodate their pain and disability.

The cases of Manuel and Jesus demonstrate the complexity of the quest to understand and effectively treat chronic pain and the need to assess the environmental context in which each pain sufferer attempts to cope with the pain and any associated disability. In the next chapter, an overview of theories of human pain perception and of chronic pain studies and treatment programs is offered to provide a picture of the current state of understanding of this complex and troublesome area of human experience.

CHAPTER 2

CHRONIC PAIN: THEORIES AND RESEARCH AND TREATMENT APPROACHES

INTRODUCTION

Textbook definitions generally define pain as an uncomfortable, unpleasant sensation related to current or impending tissue damage, which motivates the sufferer to avoid the perceived pain stimulus (Mountcastle 1974). However, there is no known physiological measure that can be relied on to vary in accordance with degree of clinical pain intensity (Elton et al. 1979; Gracely 1984). Thus, perception of nonexperimental pain intensity is a subjective experience reported to others through written, oral, or behavioral communication, and it is this communication that clinicians depend on when making diagnostic and treatment decisions. There is also a psychological response to pain, such as fear or anger; humans also attempt to attach meaning to their pain. Thus, in humans, the pain experience is a complex phenomenon involving sensory, motivational, psychological, emotional, and cognitive components.

In an attempt to provide a standard definition of human pain that recognizes its varied components, the International Association for the Study of Pain (IASP) recently defined pain as "an unpleasant sensory and emotional experience associated with actual or potential tissue damage, or described in terms of such damage" (Merskey 1986:217). The IASP stresses that pain is always subjective and that each person learns the application of the word through experiences related to injury in early life.

THE GATE-CONTROL MODEL OF PAIN PERCEPTION

The recent gate-control theory, proposed and later refined by Melzack and Wall (1965, 1970, 1983; Wall and Melzack 1984, 1989) indicates that pain perception is very complex and can be affected by past learning experiences and current attitudes. It is now clear that the once-standard specificity theory of pain, based on a model of a fixed direct-line communication system from the skin or internal organs to the brain, is insufficient for explaining many pain phenomena—including phantom limb pain, reflex sympathetic dystrophy, and causalgia. (The glossary located at the end of this book provides definitions for the medical and technical terms presented in this and other chapters.) The gate-control theory strongly suggests that complex physiological processes as well as psychological and cognitive processes (heavily influenced by sociocultural learning and experiences) affect human pain perception and response (see figure 2.1). Melzack and Wall proposed that "a gating mechanism in the dorsal horns of the spinal cord allows the perception of pain to be modified at the levels of the spinal cord, subcortex, and the cerebral cortex" (Saxon 1991:12).

A simplified discussion of the nervous system components relating to pain perception will contribute to a better understanding of the gate-control theory. Current physiological theory, which admits to being incomplete and which is constantly being further investigated and refined, suggests that the skin, muscles, and internal organs contain free nerve endings activated by stimuli that are actually or potentially harmful (Maciewicz and Sandrew 1985:17). The free nerve endings that respond to noxious stimuli are termed nociceptors. Nociceptors have no special structure designed solely to detect injury but are sensitive to noxious stimuli as well as to other properties such as heat, cold, or pressure. When nociceptors are activated by noxious stimulation, they generate impulses that are transmitted along afferent peripheral nerve fibers to the central nervous system (CNS). These free nerve endings may or may not have an insulating covering called myelin. The speed of nerve-impulse transmission to the CNS varies depending on the size of the nerve ending and the myelin status (Chapman 1984:1261).

The nerve fibers are subdivided into three major types, labeled A, B, and C fibers. Two kinds of A fibers are involved in pain perception, including the small myelinated A-delta fibers, which transmit pain signals; about 25% of these fibers respond swiftly to tissue damage stimuli, B fibers do not carry nociceptive information. C fibers (small, unmyelinated) are slow-conducting fibers, 20–50% of which respond to noxious stimulation (Chapman 1984:1261).

A-delta and C fibers, the major nocicepetors, enter the spinal cord in the back of the body and run the entire length of the spinal cord (figure 2.2). The nerve fibers enter at the dorsal horns, which consist of the first six layers of cells in the center of the spinal cord (Maciewicz and Sandrew

Figure 2.1. Gate-Control Model

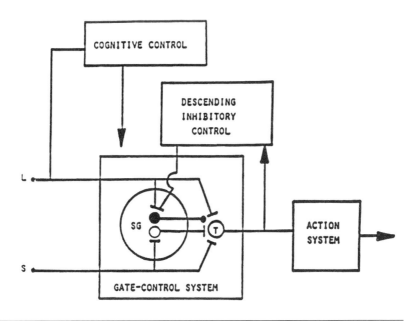

Source: Melzack and Wall, 1988.

1985; Melzack and Wall 1983). The first two layers, called the substantia gelatinosa, are where the A-delta and C fibers enter the spinal cord and connect with the central transmission nerve fibers that project to the brainstem through long-running nerve tracts (Melzack and Wall 1983; Wall and Melzack 1984) (see figure 2.3). Complex neurotransmitter substances are also involved in sensory neuron transmission (Wall and Melzack 1984).

Saxon (1991) describes neurotransmitters as "chemicals that act at the synapses between neurons and are responsible for the transmission of nerve impulses across the synaptic junctions. They may be excitatory or inhibitory" (13). At least three types of neurotransmitters are involved in pain modulation: indolamines, catecholamines, and the enkephalins/endorphins:

Indolamines, seratonin especially, seems to be related to the activity of the enkephalins/endorphins. Increasing serotonin levels in the brain results in reduced perception of pain and a higher threshold for pain, reducing serotonin level in the brain

Figure 2.2. Sensory Nerves Entering Spinal Cord

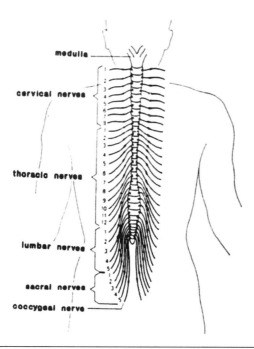

"Schematic diagram of the back of the spinal cord, showing the entering sensory nerves, the enlarged ganglia that contain the cell bodies of the nerve fibers, and the roots at the level of entry into the cord. Cervical nerves 5 and 8 and thoracic 1 aggregate on each side to form the brachial plexus which innervates each arm. Similarly, lumbar and sacral nerves form the complex lumbosacral plexus which sends nerves to the pelvis and leg." (Figure and quote from Melzack and Wall 1983:129)

increases pain perception. . . . Catecholamines (norepinephrine and dopamine, for example) also act to modify pain thresholds, lowering levels of norepinephrine in the nervous system raises the pain threshold; decreasing levels of dopamine, however, lowers the threshold for pain. . . . Enkephalin/endorphin receptors have been found in the brain, spinal cord and the gastrointestinal tract. These substances are considered to be the body's natural painkillers or morphine-like substances. Actions and interactions of the numerous and complex neurotransmitters in the nervous system as they modify and influence pain situations is a relatively new area of scientific investigation and these highly complex mechanisms are not yet clearly understood. (14)

Figure 2.3. Distribution of Nerves in Dorsal Horns

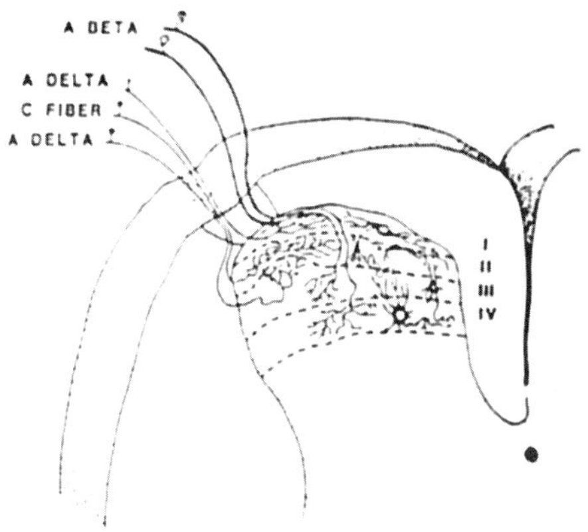

"The laminar distribution of primary afferents within the dorsal horn. Small-caliber myelinated fibers (A delta) terminate in laminae I, III and the bottom of lamina II. Unmyelinated C fibers end principally throughout lamina II, where they partially overlap the A delta input. Large diameter non-noxious cutaneous afferents enter more medially." (Figure and quote from Maciewicz and Sandrew 1985:19)

Impulses from the A-delta fibers, which are transmitted to higher areas in the brain via the relay station in the thalamus (at the top of the brainstem), result in clear, quick, well-localized and distinct pain sensations immediately associated with the injury. The C fiber activation results in slow-arriving, dull, poorly localized but persistent pain after injury (Chapman 1984:1262).

The nerve impulses arrive at the brain via two different large, long-running nerve tracts. It is currently believed that the A-delta fibers connect to the nerve fibers in the neospinothalamic tract composed of long fibers that connect to the thalamus and to a third relay of fibers that project to the sensory area of the cortex (the outer part of the brain). Information from this pathway arrives rapidly and "permits perception of the site, intensity and duration of the noxious stimuli" (Chapman 1984:1262–1264).

The C fibers apparently connect with the paleospinothalamic tract, composed of long and short fibers that project to various parts of the brain, including the thalamus, the reticular formation, and the midbrain. These pathways then connect with the forebrain and many other parts of the brain. This "paleospinothalamic pathway appears to carry information that produces motivational and emotional dimensions of the pain experience . . . and makes possible the perception of burning, aching, dull and poorly localized pain sensation" (Chapman 1984:1262).

Transmission of nerve impulses from the periphery is subject to modulation processes that can either enhance or inhibit pain transmission through various influences. These include nerve impulses descending from inhibitory pathways from the brain and pain-producing (e.g., histamine or Substance P) or pain-inhibiting (opiate) substances released by stimulation of certain nerve fibers in the CNS (Melzack and Wall 1983; Chapman 1984).

Inhibitory impulses also appear to include those from large, afferent, myelinated nerve fibers—the A-beta fibers. Wall and Melzack (1984) propose that stimulation of A-beta fibers can modulate transmission from the smaller A-delta and C fibers by activating inhibitory cells in the substantia gelatinosa of the dorsal horns (4). The *inhibitory effect* exerted by the substantia gelatinosa (SG in figure 2.1) on the afferent fiber terminals is increased by activity in the large (L) A-beta fibers and decreased by activity in small (S) A-delta and C fibers (Melzack and Wall 1983:226). This inhibitory mechanism was described by Melzack and Wall as a gate which can increase or decrease the flow of nerve impulses from peripheral nerves to the CNS; thus, somatic input may be modified *before* it evokes pain perception and response (222).

Melzack and Wall propose in addition that central control systems can inhibit pain transmission at the gates via fibers descending from the brain. Thus, cognitive or higher CNS processes such as attention, anxiety, anticipation, and memory may exert a powerful influence on the gating mechanism through the descending controls (Melzack and Wall 1983:230).

These descending transmissions are believed to arrive through corticospinal fibers from the cortex and through reticulospinal fibers from the brainstem (Melzack and Wall 1983:231). It has been determined that a high density of such nerve fiber projections runs from various areas of the brain into the substantia gelatinosa of the dorsal horns. These nerve fibers contain potentially inhibitory neurotransmitter substances such as serotonin and certain natural opiate-like substances (Maciewicz and Sandrew 1985:29–30). In addition, the brain produces morphine-like substances (endorphins), which can cause activation of spinal inhibitory processes (Chapman 1984:1264).

Many believe that there are also other descending systems as yet not clearly defined (Maciewicz and Sandrew 1985). Some possible supraspinal influences on pain perception are described in detail in Wall and Melzack (1989) and Fields and Basbaum (1989). Fields and Basbaum note that "there are probably several CNS (central nervous system) networks that modulate pain" (206). Fields and Basbaum offer an examination of evidence for analgesia produced by stimulation of certain brain sites, and for the existence of endogenous opioid peptides which provide evidence of endogenous pain-modulating systems (206). They describe one such network:

> There is a pathway that extends from the frontal cortex and hypothalamus through . . . [other brain areas to the spinal cord's] dorsal horn. . . . Activation of this system by opiates or electrical stimulation produces a selective suppression of nociceptive dorsal horn neurons and consequent analgesia. . . . [In] addition to pharmacological and surgical management of clinical pain, it may be possible to trigger pain modulating systems by psychological or physical methods . . . including suggestion. (209, 214)

The anatomy of pain perception, as visualized by Melzack and Wall and other researchers, is clearly a complex psychophysiological process involving input from various ascending and descending nerve-fiber systems and various neurotransmitter substances.

There has been widespread discussion and research regarding the gate-control theory. Garfield (1980) reports that of more than two million articles in all basic medical fields published during the 1960s, Melzack and Wall's original proposal of the gate-control theory is among the one hundred most cited papers; it is among the twelve most cited papers in the neurosciences. Many researchers have concluded that this theory is useful in addressing formerly puzzling aspects of pain; however, clinicians have been slow to act on this information (Kotarba 1983). For the most part, with the possible exception of some specialists in chronic pain, biomedical practitioners continue to employ the more traditional specificity theory of pain as a basis for diagnosis and treatment. Presumably they continue to use the specificity theory because, unlike the gate-control theory, it does not contradict the basic assumptions of the traditional biomedical paradigm, which not only divorces mental from physical states but also attributes a single symptom to a single cause (Kotarba 1983:31).

SOCIAL AND CULTURAL INFLUENCES
IN HUMAN PAIN PERCEPTION

The gate-control and other supraspinal mechanism theories propose a mind-body integration in human pain-perception processes. These theories propose that attitudes, meanings, and memories of past experiences may affect psychophysiology in such a manner that the very *perception of pain intensity* is affected (Melzack and Wall 1965; Wall and Melzack 1984, 1989; Maciewicz and Sandrew 1985; Fields and Basbaum 1989).

Attitudes, expectations, meanings for experiences, and appropriate emotional expressiveness are learned through observing the reactions and behaviors of others who are similar in identity to oneself. Obviously one's cultural or ethnic background will affect the development of meanings and attitudes. The first important source of social comparisons and learning is the family, where adults transmit to children the values and attitudes of their ethnic or cultural group (Weisenberg 1977; Sherif and Sherif 1964). Evidence of this process comes from Shorben and Borland (1954), who found that children's dental phobias were directly influenced by the attitudes of their families toward dental care. Experimental studies by Linton and Gotestam (1985), Wooley and Epps (1975), Craig and Neidermayer (1974), and Buss and Portnoy (1967) also demonstrate that social modeling and group pressure influence pain tolerance. "There is also evidence that how a person defines his or her [pain] symptoms is largely based upon consultation with family members" (Turk, Flor, and Rudy 1987:3; see also Turk and Kerns 1985; Pickens and Ireland 1969).

Further evidence of the role of family modeling and family influences in chronic pain comes from a study by Violon and Giurgea (1984), in which they compared two groups of patients as to the occurrence of chronic pain in other family members. One group consisted of chronic pain patients, the other of patients with a chronic but pain-free disease. The chronic pain group had significantly more pain patients in their families; 78% compared with 44% in the pain-free group (199). Gentry, Shows, and Thomas (1974) found that 59% of the chronic back-pain patients in their study had close family members with chronic back pain or other disabling disorders. Edwards et al. (Edwards, O'Neil, Zeichner, and Kuczmierczyk 1985; Edwards, Zeichner, Kuczmierczyk, and Boczkowski 1985) studied college students to assess the number of familial pain models available to each. They found that a substantial amount of the variance in the students' own pain complaints was predicted by the number of pain models available in their families.

After an extensive review of the literature regarding the role of the family in the etiology of chronic pain, Turk, Flor, and Rudy (1987) conclude that the observed relationships between familial pain models and the incidence of chronic pain appear to be the result of social modeling and social conditioning and learning. They note that "there is a paucity of evidence for the role of genetic variables in the development of pain problems in humans" and that it is not clear at this time how, or even if, genetic factors play a role in chronic pain problems (7).

There is, therefore, ample evidence that social learning is instrumental in the development of meanings for and attitudes toward pain. Learned values and attitudes affect one's attention to painful stimuli and one's memories of prior pain experience—factors which, according to the gate-control theory, may influence psychophysiological functioning when one is exposed to potentially painful stimuli. Since one's values, attitudes, and past social learning experiences are all influenced by enculturative experiences and ethnic/cultural background, it is obvious that one source of variation in values, attitudes, and experiences related to pain may be ethnic/cultural affiliation. A review of the literature does show that several studies of experimental and acute pain have found cultural or ethnic background to be associated with significant variation in pain intensity reports as well as attitudes, emotions, and behaviors associated with pain (Zborowski 1952, 1969; Zola 1966; Buss and Portnoy 1967; Weisenberg et al. 1975; Weisenberg et al. 1977; Knox, Shum, and McLaughlin 1977; Streltzer and Wade 1981; Lipton and Marbach 1984).

While social scientists differ regarding the precise definition of "culture," in this book culture is defined as the patterned ways that humans have learned to think about and act in their world; it involves learned, shared styles of thought and behavior which replicate the social structure of their world. As Kleinman (1988) notes, one's cultural orientation guides one's "conventional common sense about how to understand and treat illness, thus we can say of illness experience that it is always culturally shaped" (5). However, each individual's expectations regarding illness are also shaped by her or his social situation and specific life history. So despite some cultural patterning, each person has a somewhat distinct illness experience.

While cultural orientation is a component of one's ethnic heritage, ethnicity refers specifically to the condition of belonging to a particular ethnic group. An ethnic group is a *social group within a larger cultural system* which is accorded a special status (by members and nonmembers) on the basis of traits that may include, but are not limited to, religion, language, ancestry, or other historical factors. Ethnic identity refers to the individual's sense of "belonging to an ethnic group and the part of one's thinking, perceptions, feelings, and behavior that is due to ethnic group membership" (Rotheram and Phinney 1987). While ethnic-group members may share some cultural characteristics of the dominant culture, their group is unique in its worldview, and its system of values, its interactive roles, its behavioral styles, and often its language are distinctive to and shared by members (Gilbert 1989:39).

Culture thus represents the symbolic and linguistic system within which one's pain experiences are labeled and acted on (Angel and Guarnaccia 1989:1237). Clinical studies by Zborowski (1952), Lipton and Marbach (1984), Streltzer and Wade (1981), Lawlis et al. (1984), and

Greenwald (1991) all found ethnic or cultural background related to differences in reported acute pain intensity and/or responses.

However, Zborowski's and Streltzer and Wade's findings of a correlation between ethnic-group identity and differences in acute clinical pain intensity must be viewed with caution. Zborowski used only qualitative methods and failed to control for the influence of other medical, psychological, and sociocultural variables. Although Streltzer and Wade controlled for several other variables, they based their findings solely on differences in cholecystectomy patients' requests for postoperative pain medication. They did not actually measure patients' pain intensity perceptions and did not control for the influence of providers' attitudes towards requests for pain medication—which may influence patients' requests for and actual use of medication when in the hospital.

Lawlis et al. (1984) found evidence of cultural influences on pain response among chronic spinal-pain patients of Mexican American, African American, and "Caucasian" descent. They conclude that while ethnic differences were found, there was considerable intraethnic variation and the variation tended to be related to "the manner in which the pain was assessed" by the patient (751). Weaknesses of the study include the small sample size (only twenty members per group) and the lack of a standardized measure of clinical pain intensity (though a 1–100 scale was used.)

Recently, Greenwald's study of cancer patients (1991) found no statistically significant relationships between ethnic identity and measures of pain sensation, but it did find that pain described in affective terms did vary among ethnicities. However, ethnic identity was defined very loosely: the study did not exclude persons with multiple self-defined ethnic affiliations; thus, subjects could be included in multiple ethnic categories.

Lipton and Marbach's is one of the few clinical studies involving clearly defined ethnic groups and sufficient sample sizes that found statistically significant differences in pain intensity which were correlated with differences in ethnicity, with rigid controls for the influence of other variables (Lipton and Marbach 1984). They found several significant interethnic differences in pain perception in a sample of acute and chronic facial-pain patients. However, the ethnic groups did not differ on many of the variables examined. Lipton and Marbach's study also revealed differences in pain responses *within* ethnic groups, related to age and other sociodemographic variables, a finding similar to that of Lawlis et al. (1984), making it obvious that ethnicity is a complex concept and that its influence should be analyzed in a variety of ways. One major weakness of the Lipton and Marbach study is that they did not differentiate between patients with chronic pain and acute pain. This is unfortunate, because chronic pain is now recognized as a considerably different experience from acute pain.

Acute pain serves the biological function of warning the individual that something is wrong, and provides a diagnostic aid for the clinician (Leroy 1977). In contrast, chronic pain—defined as pain which continues beyond the period when it may help in detecting or healing an injury or disease, which fails to respond to usual forms of biomedical intervention, and which persists for at least three months—is now seen as a disabling disease in itself (Aronoff 1985; Fox and Melzack 1976; Kotarba 1983; Leroy 1977). Chronic pain also imposes severe physical and psychological stress (such as depression and insomnia), as well as socioeconomic hardship (severe disruption of social and work life), on the patient and family (Leroy 1977; Aronoff 1985).

In summary, existing sociological, anthropological, psychological, and medical literature reveals evidence that social learning is instrumental in the development of meanings for and attitudes toward pain. Such attitudes and ideas may well play a role in the gate-control system (through cognitive and descending inhibitory controls) and influence psychophysiological functioning upon exposure to potential painful stimuli.

Despite findings of ethnic variations in acute and experimental pain, most studies of and treatment programs for *chronic* pain (with the exception of the small study by Lawlis et al.) have ignored the possible influence of ethnic or cultural backgound on the pain experience. In addition, despite acknowledgments in the literature that cultural, psychosocial, and biological factors may interact in human illness, including chronic pain (Lawlis et al. 1984; Holzman and Turk 1986), treatment programs for chronic pain tend to focus on either the psychosocial-behavioral or the biological (Aronoff 1985; Fordyce 1976; Holzman and Turk 1986; Osterweis, Kleinman, and Mechanic 1987).

Studies also have shown that American physicians generally fail to give proper attention to cultural variation and sociocultural variables when making diagnostic and therapeutic decisions (Leiderman 1977; Kleinman, Eisenberg, and Good 1978; Good and Good 1980). As a result, when patients' cultural and socioeconomic backgrounds differ from that of the physician, often the communication between them is poor and the treatments inadequate and/or inappropriate (Weidman 1979).

If programs are to treat chronic pain sufferers successfully, it is critical that all aspects of the pain experience be better understood by both physicians and patients and that they be able to communicate effectively with each other. Despite considerable research on the psychosocial and behavioral aspects of chronic pain (Holzman and Turk 1986; Brennan et al. 1987; Dorsel 1989; Fordyce 1976; Osterweis, Kleinman, and Mechanic

1987; Good et al. 1992), and the development of chronic pain treatment programs that address psychosocial factors, all current approaches appear to ignore the influence of the *cultural* background of both patients and physicians on their relationship, their communication, and the outcome of treatment. Current treatments also ignore the ways in which patients' ethnic, cultural, or socioeconomic background shapes their chronic pain experiences and abilities to adapt successfully.

CURRENT TREATMENTS FOR CHRONIC PAIN

Despite the multidisciplinary claims of many chronic pain programs, most currently employ one of two broad approaches: (1) behavioral, cognitive, or psychological (or some combination of these three); or (2) biomedical. Very few programs combine all of these perspectives to address sociocultural, psychological, and biological factors.

Behavioral Approaches

The behavioral theoretical perspective proposes that "regardless of its source, pain eventually develops a life of its own by interacting with environmental factors that reinforce pain behavior" (Osterweis, Kleinman, and Mechanic 1987:238). Behaviorists address the problem through rehabilitation or operant conditioning programs aimed at eliminating certain "pain behaviors" (e.g., complaining; limping; staying in bed; not participating in social, recreational, and economic activities) through reinforcement of "well behaviors" and nonreinforcement of the pain behaviors (Fordyce, 1976; Osterweis, Kleinman, and Mechanic 1987; Turner and Clancy 1988). Patients' families are often also involved in a program to eliminate any "rewards" they may be providing to the patients for displaying pain behaviors. Family members are instructed in how to reward well behaviors and ignore pain behaviors.

This type of treatment is insufficient in itself, despite proponents' claims of success, for even if the pain behaviors and reports are eliminated, the perception of pain often remains (Spence 1991). Certainly, eliminating the pain behaviors has some value to the patient in terms of increased social and economic activities; however, the focus on behaviors is of equal or greater benefit to health-care providers and families, who no longer have to deal with the "deviant" pain behaviors of the sufferer. Indeed, many physicians have noted the frustrations of dealing with patients who are in pain and often angry with medical specialists who fail to help them despite repeated and costly diagnostic and treatment procedures (Osterweis, Kleinman, and Mechanic 1987; Aronoff 1985; Holzman and Turk 1986). By eliminating their patients' pain behaviors, physicians can feel a sense of success and free themselves from troublesome interactions with angry, frustrated patients. The families are often grateful as well, probably for many of the same reasons.

Chronic pain is also a major concern of government and private agencies in charge of disability programs (Osterweis, Kleinman, and Mechanic 1987). Behavioral treatments are specifically designed to reinforce well behaviors, such as vocational planning and return to work. Thus, the behavioral approach has many characteristics of a social-control mechanism. It is directed at resocialization, at eliminating deviant behaviors, and at getting the patients back to work (eliminating them from the disability rolls and counting them again as "productive" workers). Along with the social value of work, this behavioral approach mirrors American white middle-class values related to the importance of "working" on a problem, taking individual responsibility for one's actions and problems, and remaining stoic and nonexpressive in the face of pain and adversity.

This approach not only ignores differences in beliefs and values among patients of varied ethnic and cultural backgrounds, but it also places tremendous pressure on the individual patients, who are told that only by changing their own actions and attitudes can the chronic pain be effectively treated (Holzman and Turk 1986). The patients often still experience pain (Spence 1991), the source of which is no longer the focus of treatment. If unsuccessful at repressing or changing their pain behaviors, they feel guilt and a sense of personal failure.

Cognitive Approaches

Cognitive approaches focus on modifying the pain sufferers' subjective experience of pain (Turner and Clancy 1988). In a purist perspective, cognitive theory proposes that altering the cognitive experience of pain will lead to behavioral changes—that is, if the cognitive perception of pain intensity is reduced, the pain behaviors will disappear or diminish (Sternbach 1984). The focus is on identifying attitudes, beliefs, and expectations that are considered detrimental to the sufferers' experience and on altering the sufferers' interpretations of the pain sensations (Diamond and Coniam 1991:148–149): "Cognitive therapy does not ignore the experience of pain but aims to reduce the suffering that it produces in the patient by altering the way in which pain signals are interpreted by that individual." Pain sufferers are "taught to identify negative beliefs concerning pain and its effects, and to substitute these with positive thoughts and actions" (148).

Cognitive therapy often includes training in distracting oneself and redirecting the focus of attention away from the pain, redefining or relabeling the experience of pain as a different sensation, using imagery, educating the patient about the importance of cognitive processes in pain perception, and assisting the patient in challenging and changing beliefs and attitudes which are unhelpful (Pither and Nicholas 1991; Holzman and Turk 1986; Turk and Meichenbaum 1989; Turk, Meichenbaum, and Genest 1983; Turner and Clancy 1988; Diamond and Coniam 1991).

Through these cognitive techniques, some providers and researchers believe certain patients can come to feel a greater sense of control over their pain and their lives and will be able to alter their attitudes toward, perceptions of, and negative behaviors associated with their pain (Diamond and Coniam 1991). Reports of some success with cognitive approaches in mild or moderate *acute* pain have appeared in the literature, and a few reports claim at least temporary success with chronic pain (Osterweis, Kleinman, and Mechanic 1987:244; Melzack 1975; Melzack, Weisz, and Sprague 1963; Merskey and Magni 1990). However, others stress that there is "no strong evidence . . . that cognitive strategies are effective as a treatment of choice for chronic pain" (Osterweis, Kleinman, and Mechanic 1987:244; see also Linton 1982). Merskey and Magni conclude that "on the whole, it seems that cognitive therapy may have some benefit [with chronic pain], but this is still speculative" (1990:380).

Most researchers and clinicians suggest that any benefits of the cognitive approach are best attained if used in association with other interventions, such as behavioral techniques (Herman 1990:474; Osterweis, Kleinman, and Mechanic 1987; Merskey and Magni 1990; Diamond and Coniam 1991).

Psychological Approaches

The behavioral and cognitive approaches are similar to many psychological approaches in that all three view chronic pain as a psychosocial disturbance. The psychological approaches view the chronic pain, in part, as a medium for the expression of personal and interpersonal problems (Good et al. 1992:5). This view is claimed to be supported by psychiatric researchers' findings that chronic pain patients (who were studied in treatment programs) suffer from depression, irritability and anxiety (Good et al. 1992; Pilowski and Spence 1976; Swanson 1984).

Critics of this view note that these psychological patterns, which are assumed to play a causal role in the incidence of chronic pain, may simply be a normal human response to the suffering of chronic pain (Merskey 1987; Good et al. 1992). Thus critics note that these psychological patterns may represent not causal contributors, but results of the chronic pain experience. A lack of pre-chronic-pain psychological tests and data on the patients involved in these studies makes it impossible to prove whether the associated depression and anxiety are a cause of or a response to the chronic pain. Nonetheless, psychological treatment approaches generally emphasize teaching patients to solve and not avoid problems and involve psychotherapy with the patient and family and the use of psychopharmacological drugs (Aronoff 1985; Osterweis, Kleinman, and Mechanic 1987).

There are certainly reports of at least short-term changes in pain behaviors—such as increased physical activity and return to employment, reduction in medication use, and/or changes in self-reported pain perceptions—in some subjects who undergo behavioral, cognitive, and psychological treatments for chronic pain (Linton 1982; Keefe and Gill 1985; Aronoff 1985). However, long-term followup of more than twelve months is very uncommon; thus, no one knows for sure if these positive changes are retained through time, although reoccurrence of pain and readmission to pain centers have been noted (Stans et al. 1989; Keefe and Gill 1985; Malec et al. 1981; Swanson, Maruta, and Swenson 1979).

In addition, most studies lack control groups, and in pain management programs that combine modalities, such as cognitive and behavioral approaches, the various components of the program are not assessed independently, so it is unclear what components contributed to observed outcomes (Osterweis, Kleinman, and Mechanic 1987:242). Other problems with measuring outcomes of such treatment approaches include admission criteria to pain management programs, which are very selective (about one-third of those referred for evaluation are accepted); thus, "there is no way of knowing how representative of the entire pain population those persons are who participated" (242). Furthermore, study reports of efficacy often fail to differentiate between patients with different types of chronic pain and little data is available to determine if conclusions drawn for some groups apply to other groups with different types of pain (242).

In addition, the behavioral, cognitive, and psychological approaches to chronic pain all ignore or play down biological aspects of pain and focus on it as a psychosocial phenomenon. It is true that in many cases the physical abnormalities associated with the chronic pain are not clearly identified. However, this lack of a clear diagnosis may result as much from the present state of biomedical knowledge and diagnostic technology—which may not currently have the means for a correct diagnosis—as from the patients' so-called "psychosocial disorders." Yet such a possibility is often ignored in favor of the argument that if biomedicine has not found, or cannot repair, the physical abnormality associated with the chronic pain, then the pain must be mainly of psychosocial origin.

Increasingly, today's literature acknowledges that psychosocial and biological factors often interact in human diseases and illnesses, including chronic pain (Holzman and Turk 1986; Good et al. 1992). Nevertheless, many behavioral, cognitive, and psychological pain treatments (with the possible exception of some physical therapy and biofeedback/relaxation training) still ignore this interaction and address only psychosocial "disturbances" and behaviors. In fact, one of the requirements for admission to many psychological/behavioral/cognitive pain treatment programs (especially the inpatient units) is that patients must abandon the search for further biomedical diagnoses, treatments, or surgeries. Patients who are awaiting or considering specific medical, technical, or surgical interventions are excluded from admission (Stans et al. 1989:318; Turk, Meichenbaum, and Genest 1983; Pither and Nicholas 1991).

Patients are expected to adopt the attitude that only modifications in their social environment and behavioral and psychological responses will bring relief from or improvement in their chronic pain—such programs stress that the patient must become actively responsible for her or his own pain and its treatment. The practice of excluding patients who plan further biomedical treatments is based on a belief that continued medical treatments maintain the patient in a semi- or totally passive role and thus are counterproductive in encouraging greater self-reliance and ultimately detrimental to the patient and his or her treatment (Pither and Nicholas 1991:743).

My research suggests that such an assumption is not always the case. Many patients I interviewed report that they were able to gain a sense of control over their lives and pain and return to productive activities which give them substantial life satisfaction *after* biomedical treatments (such as intravenous medications, nerve blocks, or epidural steroid injections) that reduced the pain to what they defined as tolerable levels.

Biomedical Approaches

In contrast to cognitive, behavioral, and psychological approaches, biomedical diagnoses and treatments for chronic pain have focused on a disease model that views pain mainly as a symptom of tissue damage (Mountcastle 1974; Good et al. 1992). Sociocultural and psychological factors are generally considered only after diagnostic procedures fail to reveal a biological/pathological cause for the pain. In a biomedical approach, the chronic pain is reduced to "etiological 'mechanisms'; biological processes that are measured in 'objective' quantitative terms"

(Good et al. 1992:9). The focus is on pain as the result of change in material elements of the body such as "sensory receptors, afferent neuronal relays, way stations in spinal-cord, midbrain, or higher cortical modulating systems" (9). "Treatment is aimed at diminishing the neurophysiological or nociceptive aspects of the pain with traditional medical approaches. . . . [Thus, treatment is] aimed at diminishing the pain *per se*" (Pither and Nicholas 1991:744–745).

Biomedical chronic pain treatment programs are often affiliated with anesthesiology departments and may use surgery; oral or intravenous medications, including oral nonopiate analgesics, anti-inflammatories and muscle relaxants (Osterweis, Kleinman, and Mechanic 1987:241), and intravenous lidocaine[1] (Edwards, Habib et al. 1985); myofascial trigger-point injections; nerve blocks; epidural steroid injections; and transcutaneous electrical nerve stimulators (TENS) (Osterweis, Kleinman, and Mechanic 1987). Although these programs may offer nutritional counseling, physical and occupational therapy, and some psychological counseling, they often do not adequately treat the psychosocial, behavioral, and cognitive—and they generally ignore cultural—influences on the chronic pain experience. That is, they fail to address the human reality of the pain experience, which involves relationships among physiological, psychological, cognitive, socioeconomic, and cultural processes (Melzack and Wall 1965; Wall and Melzack 1989; Bates 1987; Bates and Edwards 1992; Good et al. 1992).

Because they often exclude each other, the psychological, behavioral, and cognitive approaches and the biomedical approach offer only partial treatments, and reports of improvement are often short-term; favorable results often lessen or disappear in long-term follow-up evaluations (Stans et al. 1989; Keefe and Gill 1985; Malec et al. 1981; Swanson, Maruta, and Swenson 1979). It appears that an integrated treatment model—one that conceptualizes and addresses the interaction of physiological, psychosocial, socioeconomic, and cultural influences on human pain perception and response—would be more productive and useful.

The next chapter reports on an investigation of how several particular cultural, psychosocial, socioeconomic, cognitive, biological, and health-care variables affect the human chronic pain experience.

---

1. Information on the use of lidocaine infusions in the treatment of certain types of chronic pain can be found in Edwards, Habib et al. 1985

CHAPTER 3

A NEW ENGLAND STUDY OF CULTURAL INFLUENCES ON THE CHRONIC PAIN EXPERIENCE

INTRODUCTION

Prior to my New England study, there had been very few systematic quantitative studies of the relationship of ethnic- or cultural-group affiliation to *chronic* pain perception and response. Kotarba's study (1983) of the social dimensions of chronic pain did not focus on ethnic or sociocultural variables but only on how chronic pain affects a person's behavior and relationships in social situations. Yet Kotarba has proposed that chronic pain experiences are strikingly similar across various socioeconomic and cultural groups and that a single model of the chronic pain "career" is sufficient for describing *all* chronic pain sufferers.

In light of studies demonstrating ethnic differences in response to both experimentally induced pain and acute clinical pain (Buss and Portnoy 1967; Lipton and Marbach 1984; Weisenberg et al. 1975; Weisenberg et al. 1977; Zborowski 1952), it would seem remarkable if no such differences existed among chronic pain sufferers.

The New England research design combined quantitative and qualitative methods in order to assess macro processes (wider social, political, and economic processes, such as the structure and actual function of health-care insurance, workers' compensation, and other disability systems within U.S. society, and the nature of employment conditions and power structures among various socioeconomic classes in the United States). The study also assessed micro processes (sociocultural, political, and economic relationships and processes within the immediate health-care setting, including the doctor-patient relationship, and within participants' family and social networks and individual workplaces).

In an effort to integrate a political and economic analysis with a bio-cultural perspective, a study was designed which would clarify the relationship between ethnic- or cultural-group background and variation in chronic pain perception and response while at the same time assessing and statistically controlling for the effects of other biological, psychosocial, and socioeconomic variables on the complex process of human adaptation to the chronic pain experience. Using qualitative methods, an attempt was also made to clarify the political, economic, and cultural context in which care, treatment, compensation, and rehabilitation are provided (or denied), and to assess the impact of that context on patients' chronic pain experiences.

The definition of adaptation to chronic pain used in the studies reported on in this book was arrived at after initial interviews with the case-study patients in the New England study (and later supplemented by other case-study interviews with island Puerto Rican participants) and is based on an emic (or subject's) point of view. After discussing what criteria numerous participants used to define effective coping and adjustment, and while acknowledging the ever-changing nature of chronic pain, I define positive adaptation to chronic pain as an ongoing process of adjusting behaviors and attitudes in order to manage the pain, disability, and associated uncertainty and continue a life defined by the subject as meaningful and worthwhile. In the New England and Puerto Rican studies, successful adaptation (as defined by the subjects' themselves) was associated with a reduction in or ability to overcome temporary bouts of depression, unhappiness, fear, and worry; the realistic resumption and continuation of family, social, and work roles; and the recognition and acceptance of unalterable limitations.

In contrast, negative adaptations included drug dependency, a constant unrealistic search for an external "cure," and a reluctance or refusal to engage in activities one is capable of doing. Participants reported that these strategies were often associated with severe depression, anger, fear, worry, and/or unhappiness.

In the analyses reported on in this book, level of adaptation was ultimately assessed using the following four criteria: (1) effective use of biomedical and other health-care resources, including use (without overuse) of medications (for example, controlling frequency and dosage of medications to lessen long-term side effects), biomedical services, and nonbiomedical healers and methods; (2) behavioral adjustment and functioning, including mobility and engagement in activities of daily living; (3) psychological adjustment and functioning, including degree of depression, anger, worry, happiness, and overall life satisfaction; and (4) cognitive adjustments such as acceptance of limits of illness without either denial or undo catastrophizing.

THE STUDY POPULATION

The New England study was conducted at a pain control center in New England during 1987 and 1988. The pain center is an outpatient multidisciplinary chronic pain treatment facility founded in 1976. The clinic is part of an anesthesiology department at the medical center where it is located. The clinic literature states that it uses a "multidisciplinary" approach to achieve its stated goals: (1) reduce the amount of pain experienced by the patient as much as possible; (2) increase the patient's understanding and awareness of what causes the pain; (3) improve the lifestyle and day-to-day functioning of the patient; and (4) help the patient get back to work if currently not working.

All patients are seen and treated by the clinic's medical doctors (specialists in anesthesiology and chronic pain), who use various treatments, including nerve blocks, intravenous lidocaine infusions, trigger-point injections, epidural steroid injections, and, for the most part, nonopiate prescription medications. The staff discourages long-term reliance on opiate drugs; however, short-term use is not uncommon, and many new patients who are narcotic-dependent upon arrival are put on methadone, which is then decreased gradually.

Each patient is given a battery of psychological tests and is seen by one of the clinic's psychologists for an initial evaluation and, if deemed necessary by the clinic physicians, for further treatment. If appropriate, patients are also treated by nutritionists; physical and occupational therapists; biofeedback, behavior modification, and relaxation specialists; and other medical specialists such as neurologists or orthopedists.

The clinic was chosen for the research for several reasons. First, to meet the goals of the New England study it was absolutely essential to study the chronic pain experience in a nonlaboratory setting among actual chronic pain sufferers. The clinic has a large outpatient population with approximately six thousand patient visits per year (many patients come for repeat weekly or biweekly treatments). Such a large patient population allowed for adequate sample sizes for valid statistical analyses.

Secondly, while admittedly only a broad estimator of ethnic variability, United States census data for 1980 indicated considerable ethnic diversity in the city where the pain center is located (Bureau of the Census 1980). Ethnic identification was further clarified in this city by the presence of localized ethnic neighborhoods and churches. In addition, an early meeting with the director and head nurse at the clinic revealed that, while no specific questions on ethnic identity had been asked on clinic screening materials, the staff had noted considerable ethnic variability in the patient population.

Finally, the clinic collects a great deal of sociodemographic, psychological, and medical-history data, as well as several measures of pain intensity and response, from all patients when they enter the clinic. These data were made available so the patients would not have to be asked to complete numerous lengthy questionnaires.

The study was reviewed and granted approval by the Committee on the Protection of Human Subjects in Research at the Medical Center, and informed consent was obtained from each participant.

All patients who participated in this study were defined as having *chronic* pain by the pain center physicians. The criteria used to define chronic pain in this study were based on guidelines set by the International Association for the Study of Pain (IASP) as suggested in the Classification of Chronic Pain (Merskey 1986). The IASP-suggested point of division between acute and chronic pain of 3 months (Merskey 1986:S5) was used as the minimum duration standard for inclusion in this study. Other IASP criteria for chronic pain in the study included pain that persisted past the expected normal time of healing and that failed to respond to usual forms of biomedical intervention (Bonica 1985; Wall and Melzack 1984, 1989; Merskey 1986). The range for pain duration in this study population was 3 months to 504 months, with a population mean of 50 months.

The pain center's chronic pain patient population consisted of members of twenty-eight ethnic groups. Ethnic identity was determined with an Ethnicity and Pain Survey devised for this study, which determined language and religion in the patient's childhood home; birth place of patient, parents, and grandparents; and patient's primary ethnic-group self-identification (see appendix A). All patients who reported more than one primary ethnic affiliation were eliminated from the project, so that the study analyzed only discrete ethnic groups.

The six largest ethnic/cultural groups at the pain center were included in the study. The first group comprised Anglo Americans (N = 100); they were generally at least third-generation U.S.-born patients who identified themselves with no ethnic group; the majority were Protestants. This is a category first defined by Zborowski (1952) and referred to by him as "Old Americans." His observation at that time still appears accurate today: "the values and attitudes of this group dominate in the country and are held by [many] members of the medical profession" (19). At the pain center, members of this group defined themselves first as Americans and often mentioned a secondary self-identification as a "Yankee" or "New Englander." The other groups in the pain center study were Latinos (N = 44), Irish (N = 60), Italians (N = 50), French Canadians

(N = 90), and Polish (N = 28). All of the chronic pain patients treated at the pain center during the study period who identified one of these six groups as their sole primary affiliation were approached and asked to participate in the study. Of the 438 patients asked to participate, 85% (N = 372) agreed.[1]

According to the Census Bureau, the major ancestry groups in the city where the study was conducted and in the surrounding congressional district (which has a total population of 521,949) are French (65,934), Polish (35,245), Irish (34,148), English (33,457), Black American (27,594), Italian (25,918), and Latino or "of Spanish origin" (19,086) (Bureau of the Census 1980). Thus, the six groups in the study population reflect the region's predominant ancestral groups, with the exception of Black Americans. Only seven Black Americans were encountered in the patient population during the study period, obviously too small a group to include in the analysis.

Characteristics of the study population are presented in table 3.1.

METHODS AND PROCEDURES

The major research questions which the *quantitative* segment of the pain center study sought to answer were:

(1) What, if any, cultural, sociodemographic, psychological, and biological variables are associated with statistically significant differences in reported pain intensity and pain responses in the pain center population?

(2) Are there statistically significant differences in reported pain intensity and pain responses in the pain center population which are related to ethnic identity, when other sociodemographic, psychological, and biological variables are controlled?

––––––––––

1. The characteristics of the New England patients who refused to participate are unknown because I did not have access to the medical records of those who refused. In accordance with the procedures for the protection of human subjects at the New England medical center and, as stated in the project consent form, written permission had to be granted before review of patients' records. Thus, I cannot determine the sociodemographic or medical characteristics of those who refused. The New England patients who refused were asked to participate in person when they visited the clinic or were sent a written request to participate and did not respond. I can report that all those who refused in person said they did so because of pending workers' compensation cases or other litigation cases and despite assurances that confidentiality would be maintained. However, many others involved in such cases agreed to participate.

Table 3.1. Characteristics of the New England Study Population

Charac-teristic	Anglo American	Latino	Italian	French Canadian	Irish	Polish	F-ratio	Sig.
			Ethnic Groups					
Age							1.0	.42
Mean	43.5	41.2	46.6	44.3	46.2	46.7		
SD	14.7	10.5	15.9	14.7	15.7	15.5		
Education[a]							12.8	.00*
Mean	12.7	8.7	11.3	11.8	12.5	13.1		
SD	2.8	3.4	3.1	2.9	3.1	2.2		
No. of Medications							1.5	.19
Mean	2.1	2.3	2.3	2.1	2.3	2.1		
SD	1.6	1.7	1.7	1.5	1.6	1.4		
Duration[b]							.5	.81
Mean	49.7	54.1	48.7	49.9	57.3	35.9		
SD	63.9	56.1	82.6	60.7	66.0	39.8		
							Chi-square	Sig.
Gender							5.9	.32
Male	50	29	28	42	35	14		
Female	50	15	21	48	25	14		
Religion							53.2	.00*
Catholic	32	30	39	61	42	25		
Protest.	44	11	3	15	11	2		
Workers' Comp.							2.7	.74
Yes	33	22	20	36	24	12		
No	55	20	24	46	31	16		
Diagnosis							14.8	.14
Low-Back Pain[c]	53	27	31	43	23	15		
Neuritis, etc.[d]	8	0	2	15	7	3		
Arthritis	3	3	2	3	7	1		

SD = Standard Deviation

*$p < .05$

[a] Total years of education.

[b] Duration is in number of months in pain.

[c] Low-back pain = radicular, mechanical, and postsurgical low-back and herniated and degenerative discs.

[d] Neuritis, neuralgia, and other neuropathies.

(3) Are there statistically significant intra-ethnic-group variations in pain intensity and responses within any of the pain center ethnic groups; and, if so, what variables are associated with those intragroup differences?

The independent variables in the *quantitative component* of the study included the cultural, sociodemographic, psychological, and medical variables which other studies indicated may be related to variation in human pain perception and response (Zborowski 1952, 1969; Zola 1966; Weisenberg et al. 1975; Wright et al. 1983; Lawlis et al. 1984; Lipton and Marbach 1984; Sargent 1986, 1989). These variables were ethnic-group affiliation, degree of heritage consistency (defined by Estes and Zitzow [1980] and Spector [1985] as the degree to which one's lifestyle reflects one's traditional culture) and patient's generation; sociodemographic variables including age, gender, current religion, and socioeconomic status (SES) as determined by education, occupation, and household income; workers' compensation status; the cognitive/psychological orientation known as locus-of-control (LOC) style; and medical variables reflecting types and number of previous surgeries, types and number of previous pain treatments, types and number of current medications for pain, and clinical diagnosis associated with the chronic pain.

The first dependent variable in the quantitative analysis was the reported perception of pain intensity as measured by the McGill Pain Questionnaire (MPQ). The MPQ has been widely employed to measure human pain and is often included in preliminary assessment materials of chronic pain treatment facilities, including those of the pain center. The MPQ was subjected to intense validity testing by Melzack and Torgenson (1971) prior to its widespread distribution. During this testing a high degree of agreement on the intensity relationships among the MPQ's pain descriptors was obtained from subjects who had different cultural, socio-economic, and educational backgrounds (Melzack 1984:335). The MPQ has also been employed in over sixty published studies of pain (Turk, Rudy, and Salovey 1985; Gaston-Johansson et al. 1985). Because of its reliability, availability, and widespread use, the MPQ was utilized in the pain center study to measure reported pain intensity.

The MPQ is made up of seventy-eight words which describe pain; it is divided into three major categories—sensory, affective and evaluative. The words are arranged into twenty subclasses, each of which is contained in a single box on the questionnaire (see appendix B). The patient chooses the one word in each subclass that best describes his or her pain. The words chosen may be analyzed in two ways: (1) the total number of words chosen in a major category, and (2) a pain rating index (PRI) based on the numerical values assigned to the chosen words.

In the PRI scoring system, the words in each subclass are given numerical values: the first word in each subclass, which implies the least pain, is given a value of 1; the next word is given a value of 2; the next 3; and so on. The values of the words chosen in each major category are then added up to give a total for the category. All categories are also totaled to give a pain intensity grand total score which is referred to as the pain rating index total (MPQ-PRIT). The MPQ-PRIT is currently considered one of the best measures of overall pain severity (Melzack and Torgenson 1971; Melzack 1975, 1984; Elton et al. 1979; Gracely 1984; Turk, Rudy, and Salovey 1985). This study assessed the MPQ-PRIT and also the sensory and affective subcategories of the MPQ to determine if there was ethnic variation in these sub-areas as well.

An attempt was made to select, as far as possible, measurement instruments that have been found valid for use with Latino and non-Latino Caucasian populations. The MPQ has been extensively used internationally (languages include English, French, Swedish, and Spanish) for the assessment of acute and chronic pain (Fox and Melzack 1976; Fotopoulos, Graham, and Cook 1979; Prieto et al. 1980; Lahuerta, Smith, and Martinez-Lage 1982; Molina, Coppo, and del Dorente 1984). The Latino patients at the pain center who spoke only Spanish were given a Spanish version of the MPQ during the study period, as it was not available at the pain center until it was introduced as part of this project (see appendix B for English and Spanish versions of the MPQ).

The other dependent variables involved a variety of responses to the chronic pain, including behavioral responses such as changes in work and social activities; degree of expressiveness of pain, including verbal and body language expressions; psychological responses such as anger, fear, and depression; and attitudinal responses such as belief in the ability to overcome the pain and attitudes towards pain and the ability to lead a happy and productive life.

The final dependent variable was adaptation to the chronic pain, which, as noted earlier, involves the ongoing process of adjustment in behavior and attitudes that facilitates resumption and continuation of a life defined by the pain sufferer as meaningful and worthwhile. Adaptation was determined by questions on the Ethnicity and Pain Questionnaire, the pain center's admission questionnaire, and through formal and informal interviews and observations.

Information on patients' cultural and sociodemographic backgrounds and pain responses and experiences was obtained from the Ethnicity and Pain Survey and an Ethnicity and Pain Questionnaire, also devised for this study (see appendix C for the Ethnicity and Pain Questionnaire).

The Ethnicity and Pain Questionnaire questions are worded in statement form, with response selections based on a Likert-type scale: (0) not applicable, (1) disagree somewhat, (2) disagree strongly, (3) agree somewhat, and (4) agree strongly. This scale is often used as an interval measure in social science studies of medical or psychological populations (Lipton and Marbach 1984; Guagnano et al. 1986), as it is here.

The Ethnicity and Pain Questionnaire also includes questions to assess the psychological/cognitive style known as locus-of-control (LOC), because numerous studies have found a relationship between LOC style and variation in ways of coping with or responding to stressful life events, including illness and pain (Rotter 1966; Lefcourt 1980; Coreil and Marshall 1982; Kist-Kline and Lipnickey 1989; Afflek et al. 1987; Buckelew et al. 1990). When viewed as ideal types, an internal LOC style involves a reported cognitive perception or expectation that life events and circumstances are the result of one's own actions, whereas an external LOC style includes the perception or expectation that life events and circumstances are beyond one's own control, in the hands of fate, chance, or other people (Coreil and Marshall 1982).

When selecting the items from Rotter's original LOC scale (1966) to be used in the Ethnicity and Pain Questionnaire, the items pertaining to luck/fate and leadership/success were chosen because those dimensions have shown adequate cross-cultural equivalence when used with non-Latino Caucasian and Latino populations (Garza and Widlak 1977). The questions from Rotter's scale that pertain to academies, politics, and respect were omitted because their validity for Latino populations is seriously in question (Garza and Widlak 1977). Five of the ten true/false LOC items on the Ethnicity and Pain Questionnaire are worded in an internal direction, indicating a sense of personal control, and five are worded in an external direction. Following a scoring practice described by Tait, Chibnall, and Richardson (1982), internally worded items are reverse-scored; thus, a high total score on the ten items indicates an external LOC tendency, and a low total score reflects internal LOC expectancies. Following a practice described by Krause and Stryker (1984), internal and external LOC groups were categorized by splitting the LOC scores at the total study-population mean: those above the mean fall into the external group and those at and below the mean fall into the internal group.

The Ethnicity and Pain Questionnaire questions used to determine degree of heritage consistency were adapted from the work of Estes and Zitzow (1980) and Spector (1985) and asked if the participants: (1) were born and raised in the ethnic group's country of origin or in an ethnic neighborhood, (2) lived in an ethnic neighborhood as adults, (3) maintained regular contact with their extended family and engaged primarily in social activities with members of their ethnic group, (4) had knowledge of and pride in the culture and language of their origin, and (5) felt the traditional heritage still played an important role in their present lifestyle. According to Spector (1985), a high aggregated score on these questions indicates strong ties to one's group or a high degree of heritage consistency (and a correspondingly lower degree of assimilation or acculturation to the culture of the dominant group).

Many other questions on the Ethnicity and Pain Questionnaire were adapted from Lipton and Marbach's study (1984), because their questions were carefully constructed from statements often made by pain sufferers about their own pain experiences and verified by physicians who treat pain sufferers. (Some rewording of the questions was necessary, as Lipton and Marbach studied only facial-pain patients and often phrased their questions in terms of facial pain only.) Before use at the pain center, the Ethnicity and Pain Questionnaire was pretested—with a group of chronic pain sufferers attending a back-pain school at a university-affiliated health center (not the pain center)—to verify that its statements were relevant to the experiences of chronic pain patients.

The Ethnicity and Pain Survey was completed by all new patients before their first visit; it was given to other patients in person or by mail. The Ethnicity and Pain Questionnaire was usually administered in a personal interview during the patients' regularly scheduled visits or by mail or phone when in-person interviews could not be arranged. Latino patients not fluent in English were interviewed in Spanish (see appendix D for the Spanish Ethnicity and Pain Questionnaire). Data were also collected from patients' medical records and the pain center's admission questionnaire (see appendix E) and files.

The pain center data also included a psychological evaluation by a clinic psychologist for each patient (with the exception of Latinos who did not speak or read English—no psychological tests or services were offered in Spanish).

Statistical analysis, using the SPSSx Information Analysis System, was conducted at the Social and Demographic Research Institute at the University of Massachusetts at Amherst. The analyses included F-tests, Student-t tests, chi-squares, Pearson Correlation Coefficients, and multiple regression analysis. Alpha was set at .05. Characteristics of the six ethnic groups were compared by one-way analysis of variance (ANOVA) for each of the independent variables.

Qualitative Methods: In addition to the quantitative data collection and analyses, numerous formal and informal interviews were conducted with many of the patients at the pain center—during these interviews open-ended questions were asked. Six patients were also selected from each of the six ethnic groups from whom intensive case-study materials were gathered. I chose case-study patients who represented the range of age, gender, diagnoses, pain duration, and LOC styles in each group. The case-study patients were interviewed on several occasions in addition to the initial interview, which elicited the quantitative information. All intensive case-study interviews were conducted at the pain center. In addition to the formal case-study interviews, many patients came in for weekly treatments involving procedures that lasted one to three hours, so I was able to visit with and/or observe many of the case-study participants on a weekly or biweekly basis throughout most of the pain-center study period. The majority of case-study patients preferred that interviews not be tape recorded, so notes were taken during the interviews and extensive fieldnotes were recorded at the completion of each case-study interview as well as after each informal encounter with case-study patients.

I also talked informally with many relatives of patients in the waiting room. I recorded observations of patients, relatives, and the staff on a daily basis. I also attended and recorded fieldnotes on several of the weekly staff meetings in which certain patients' cases were evaluated or reevaluated by the pain center staff of physicians, psychologists, occupational and physical therapists, and nurses. I also observed and recorded information on changes in staffing and, when the New England center's nursing and medical staffs were reduced by the administration, I obtained interview data on why the cuts had been made and on how staff reacted to these cuts. I continually observed and recorded data on medical and support staffs' behaviors, and on my informal and formal talks and interviews with them.

In addition, I was present during many procedures, including installing of IV lines for intravenous medications; during patients' recovery periods from other procedures, such as rest periods following administration of epidural steroids; and I observed many exchanges between nurses, doctors, psychologists, occupation therapists, and other staff concerning treatment and rehabilitation decisions and their assessment of patients' response to treatment plans and actual treatment.

I also observed numerous encounters between physicians, nurses, and other staff and patients and their relatives. Especially noteworthy were observed encounters with patients who did not have appointments but who had come to the center seeking physicians' evaluations for their compensation or disability-related paperwork. Often doctors had failed to complete such paperwork which patients had previously left with them during earlier scheduled visits. Many patients returned to attempt face-to-face encounters with physicians to elicit the doctors' assistance with required paperwork as deadlines approached.

Through these processes of observation and data collection, I recorded patterns of health-care providers' decision making and the values, beliefs, and attitudes expressed by providers. I also recorded providers' expressed views of their patients and patients' responses to care and treatment and the providers' views on workers' compensation and other disability compensation issues. These data were used to conceptualize and analyze the nature of biomedical culture at the pain control center. Thus, a major goal of the qualitative data collection was to define the political, economic, and sociocultural context in which treatment, compensation, and rehabilitation are provided to chronic pain patients and to assess the impact of that context on patients' chronic pain experiences.

*Sociodemographic and Cultural Characteristics
of the Study Population*

The Latinos were the most recent arrivals to the New England area; 35 of 44 members were born outside the U.S. mainland, 34 in Puerto Rico and one in Costa Rica. Most of these non-U.S.-mainland-born patients had moved to the area within the previous five years. The majority of the Latino group (33 out of 44) did not speak English fluently as adults. The majority of the members of the Polish (21 of 28) and Italian (30 of 50) groups were members of the first or second generation in their families to be born in the United States, and many spoke English as well as Polish or Italian as adults. The majority of the members of the Irish group (42 of 60) and of the French Canadian group (55 of 90) were members of the second, third, or greater generation in their families to be born in the United States; many of the French Canadians spoke both English and French as adults, while most of the Irish spoke only English as adults, although several reported speaking Gaelic in their childhood home (see figure 3.1 for generation distributions.)

As figure 3.2 indicates, the Latino, Italian, and Polish groups had the highest means on the heritage consistency section of the Ethnicity and Pain Questionnaire, indicating that members of these groups felt the strongest ties to their ethnic groups and had lifestyles which most strongly reflected their traditional ethnic culture ($F = 4.94$, $p < .01$). A Duncan's Multiple Range Test showed that the significant differences in heritage-consistency means appeared between the Anglo American

Figure 3.1. Generation Distributions

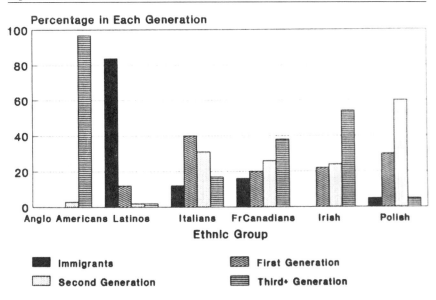

Figure 3.2. Heritage Consistency Means

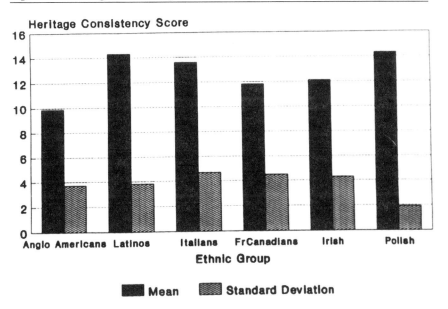

group (which had the lowest mean of 9.9) and each of the other five groups and between the Latino group (which had the highest mean of 14.3) and both the French Canadian and Irish groups.

As indicated in table 3.1, there were no significant differences among the six groups in mean age, gender distributions, household income levels, and workers' compensation status. The Latino group had a significantly lower mean for years of education than the other five groups.

The major differences in occupational distributions were between the Latino group and the other five groups and between the Italian group and both the Polish and Irish groups (chi-square = 41.9, $p < .01$). The occupations were categorized as: no-salaried occupation (housewives, students, and never-employed persons), unskilled workers, semiskilled workers, skilled workers, and professionals. The Latino group had a higher percentage of members in the unskilled, semiskilled, and no-salaried occupations than did the other five groups. In each of the other five groups, the skilled category held the highest number of people; in contrast, in the Latino group the unskilled category was largest. Another notable difference was that the Polish and Irish groups had a significantly higher percentage of members in the professional group than did the Italians. In the Italian group only 9% were professionals, while 23% of the Polish group and 26% of the Irish were professionals (figure 3.3). Finally, as indicated in table 3.1, there was a significant difference between the Anglo Americans and the other five groups in current religion. The Anglo American group was the only one with more Protestants than Catholics.

MEDICAL CHARACTERISTICS OF
THE STUDY POPULATION

There was no significant difference in the mean number of months in pain among the six groups (table 3.1). The majority of patients in all groups had some type of chronic low-back pain—mechanical, radicular, postsurgical, or degenerative or herniated disks.[2] There were no significant differences in the distribution of the most common diagnostic categories (table 3.1), these being low-back pain, arthritis, and a category composed of those with neuritis, neuralgia, or other neuropathies. There were no significant differences in the distribution of the most common past treatments for

---

2. Low-back pain is a commonly used generic diagnostic category for chronic pain patients whose pain is viewed as having disc-related or musculoskeletal etiology (Flor and Turk 1989).

Figure 3.3. Occupational Distributions

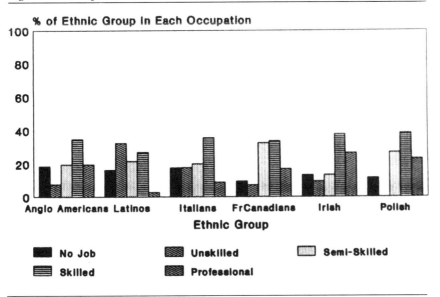

pain, which included chiropractic, use of transcutaneous electrical nerve stimulators (TENS), nerve blocks, and physical therapy. Nor were there significant differences in the mean number of medications or in the distributions of medication types being taken for pain. The five most commonly used medication classes were nonopiate analgesics, opiate analgesics, anti-depressants, anti-inflammatory drugs, and muscle relaxants.

COGNITIVE STYLES/PSYCHOLOGICAL CHARACTERISTICS OF PAIN CENTER POPULATION

A significant relationship was found between LOC style and ethnic identity (figure 3.4), as there was a significant difference in the distribution of the two styles across the ethnic groups (chi-square = 22.52, $p < 0.01$). In the Latino group over 80% reported an external LOC style. In contrast, 90% of the members of the Polish group were in the internal subgroup, as were approximately 60% of the French Canadian group and 65% of the Italian and Irish groups. In the Anglo American group, 50% were in the external and 50% in the internal subgroup.

Thus, except for the Anglo American group, ethnic identity was a predictor of LOC style. As it is impossible for LOC style to influence ethnic identity, probably ethnic background (i.e., socialization and psychoso-

Figure 3.4. LOC Style Distributions by Ethnicity

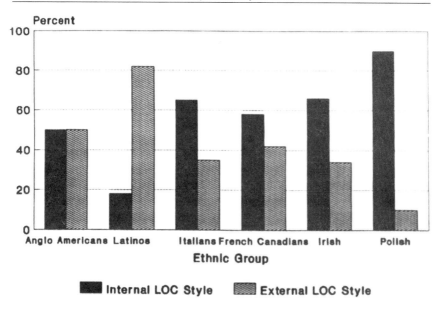

cial experiences as a member of the group) has an effect on the LOC style one is most likely to develop.

Several researchers have noted that Latin American cultural tradition views reality as uncontrollable rather than as something that can be manipulated or transformed (Sanchez-Ayendez 1984; Bastida 1979). In this worldview, although humans can control certain aspects of their physical and social environments and their lives, they can never completely dominate nature or their environment. North American social scientists have seen this as a passive and pessimistic attitude, although Latino and Latin American researchers view it as realistic (Bastida 1979:43–58; Sanchez-Ayendez 1984:64–65; Duany 1988–89). Latino researchers note that Latinos often accept that there are aspects of life that are disagreeable, and they openly admit one might not desire certain aspects such as sickness and death (Sanchez-Ayendez 1984). In addition, Ghali (1982) has noted that the history of Puerto Rico's colonization, the island's eventual industrialization (which displaced many agricultural workers), as well as the island's current nebulous political status, have left many island and mainland Puerto Ricans with a sense of powerlessness (98). These historical and current political, social, and economic realities and the Latin American cultural orientation toward reality may help explain why more New England Latinos, who are mostly immigrants from Puerto Rico, fall into the external LOC style than do members of the non-Latino groups.

There were no significant relationships between the distribution of the two LOC styles and the other sociodemographic variables in this study, including age, gender, SES, and religion.

In summary, the six ethnic groups in this study were similar in many respects; for example, there were no statistically significant differences among the groups in mean age, gender distributions, household income levels, workers' compensation status, marital status, mean pain duration, mean numbers of current medications for pain, or distributions of the types of pain medication being taken, types of past pain treatments, or major diagnostic categories. The major differences among the groups were limited to LOC-style distributions, education level (with the only significant difference being between the Latino group and the other five groups), and religion (with the Anglo Americans being the only group with more Protestants than Catholics). Thus, the study population offered the opportunity for a comparison of the chronic pain experiences of members of six ethnic groups which exhibit very few statistically significant differences in sociodemographic and medical characteristics.

CHAPTER 4

VARIATIONS IN REPORTED PAIN INTENSITY IN THE NEW ENGLAND POPULATION

Studies of health and illness indicate that different cultural or ethnic groups often have dissimilar health beliefs and standards for illness behaviors (Jordan 1993; Lipton and Marbach 1984; Mechanic 1972; Zborowski 1952). While there is a range of variation within any cultural group related to factors such as age, gender, individual personality, or family environment, studies show that members of various groups often perceive, label, respond to, and communicate symptoms differently and make different health-care choices (Lipton and Marbach 1984:1279).

Clinical studies of experimental and acute pain provide evidence that one's cultural background influences how one communicates, expresses, and responds to pain (Lipton and Marbach 1984; Sternbach 1974; Craig 1983; Chapman 1984). It should be stressed that this does not mean that all people from a similar background express or respond to pain in exactly the same way, but rather that cultural background can affect variation in pain response.

The effect of cultural background on *chronic* pain response is less well understood. Also, the influence of cultural-group identity on both acute and chronic pain *perception* in regard to *pain intensity* has been given inadequate attention or, when studied, has not been carefully documented using standardized assessment instruments that can be easily replicated. The research at the pain center focused on these neglected areas.

INTER-ETHNIC-GROUP PAIN INTENSITY DIFFERENCES

In the pain center study, to determine inter-ethnic-group differences in reported pain intensity, an analysis of variance (ANOVA) was performed for reported chronic pain intensity, as measured by the MPQ, by ethnic group. Similar ANOVAs were also performed for groups classified on the basis of each of the independent sociodemographic, medical, cognitive, and psychological variables. For those items showing significant F-ratio values on the ANOVA, the Duncan's Multiple Range test was also performed to determine which of the groups differed from each other for each item.

As measured by the MPQ-PRIT, reported pain intensity showed statistically significant differences associated with variation in age cohort, ethnic-group affiliation, and locus-of-control (LOC) style (figure 4.1). The age cohort composed of patients over the age of 60 had the lowest reported pain intensity mean of 28; the middle-aged cohort (ages 41–60) had the highest mean of 34; and the youngest group (20–40 years) had a mean of 32 ($F = 3.05, p < .05$).

As for differences in pain intensity among the six ethnic groups ($F = 4.08, p < .01$), the mean of the Latino group was 40, the highest of all six groups, while the Italian group mean of 32 was second highest. In contrast, the Polish and French Canadian groups had means of 29.2 and 29.3. The Anglo American and Irish groups had intermediate means of 30 and 31. A Duncan's Multiple Range test determined that the significant difference in the ANOVA was between the Latino group and each of the other five groups.

There were also significant intergroup differences in the MPQ's affective and sensory categories which were consistent with the findings for total pain intensity (MPQ-PRIT) in that the Latino group's means in both the sensory and affective categories were the highest of all six groups, the Italian group's means in both categories ranked second highest, and the Polish group had the lowest mean in the sensory category and the second to lowest (above the French Canadian group) in the affective category. (For those interested in reviewing the tables for ethnic differences in the sensory and affective categories of the MPQ, they are located in appendix F, table F.1).

In terms of the third independent variable—LOC style—the external group had a total-pain-intensity mean of 36.9, while the internal group had a significantly lower mean of 30.4 ($F = 6.86, p < 0.01$).

Appropriate statistical analyses showed that the only other independent variables related to variation in total pain intensity variation were number (but not type) of past treatments for pain, and current number (but again not type) of pain medications being taken.

Some studies suggest that the long-term use of opiate analgesics may actually increase pain intensity as well as create a drug dependency in chronic pain patients, and therefore many pain treatment programs—

Figure 4.1. Intensity Means by Age, LOC, and Ethnicity

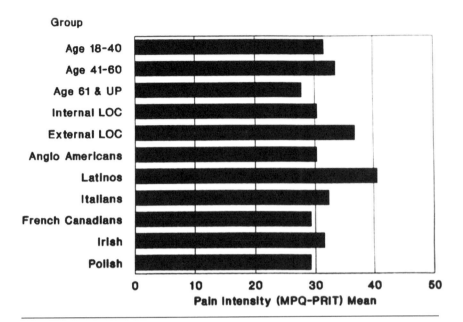

including the pain center program—involve eliminating opiate drug use (Aronoff 1985). However, the ANOVA showed that variation in total pain intensity in this study population was not significantly associated with medication types. Thus, in this population, it is likely that number of current medications was an effect rather than a cause of pain-intensity variation, as the group taking five or more medications had the highest pain-intensity mean, the group taking only one medication had the lowest pain-intensity mean, and with each additional medication the mean pain intensity increased.

Similarly, *type* of treatment was not significantly related to pain-intensity variation; however, *number* of treatments was. The relationship between number of treatments and pain intensity is most likely one in which seeking numerous treatments is a response to high pain intensity.

Appropriate statistical tests showed that the following medical variables were not related to variation in pain intensity: diagnosis, type or number of previous surgeries for pain, type of previous treatments for pain, and type of current pain medication. Because the majority of patients in the study were taking at least two medications for pain (population mean was 2.25), the MPQ-PRIT means for the most common single medications and for the most common combinations were compared, and no significant relationships were found. It must be stressed that this does not indicate that there is no biological component to the chronic pain in members of this population. While intensity *variation* was not significantly related to the medical variables, the vast majority of the patients in this study had a medical diagnosis involving physical pathology associated with the chronic pain. In addition, while significant variation in pain intensity occurred across ethnic, age, and LOC-style groups, those individuals with the lowest intensity within those groups were not pain free. Thus, members of this population have a certain degree of pain that is not subject to the variation.

Finally, gender, marital status, religion, income, occupation, education, and workers' compensation status were not significantly associated with variation in total pain intensity. Given the three major variables—ethnic identity, LOC style, and age—related to statistically significant variation in reported pain intensity, multiple regression analysis was used to examine their relationships.

As ethnic group and LOC style are qualitative, they were treated as dummy variables. (LOC style was used as a qualitative variable so that I could compare differences in intensity between the internal and external LOC-style groups. Raw LOC scores were used only to place patients into the internal or external group as described in chapter 3). Because of the interaction of LOC style and ethnic affiliation (discussed below), and a need to control for the different effects of LOC styles on pain intensity within the Anglo American and Polish groups, an interaction term for each of those two groups was included in the regression equation. Since the Latino group had the highest intensity mean, it was used as the constant for ethnicity in the regression analysis.

In the regression analysis, ethnic-group identity and LOC style remained significantly associated with pain-intensity variation after controlling for the influence of age and of each other. Age did not remain significant when ethnicity and LOC style were controlled (appendix F, table F.2). This analysis showed that 22% (R-square = .2205) of the variation in intensity was explained by the variation in age, ethnic identity, and LOC style. When other significant variables were controlled, there was a significant difference in the regression between the Latino group and the Anglo American, French Canadian, and Polish groups. While the differences between the Latino group and both the Italian and Irish groups were significant in the F-ratio analysis using the Duncan's Multiple Range test, those differences did not remain significant in the regression analysis when other variables were controlled (appendix F, table F.2).

Obviously, pain intensity cannot influence one's ethnic identity; thus, the association between reported pain intensity and ethnic identity suggests that experiences, beliefs, attitudes, and meanings derived from growing up within a particular social community may affect one's perception and/or reports of pain intensity.

INTRA-ETHNIC-GROUP PAIN INTENSITY VARIATION

A very similar pattern of cultural and LOC-style influences was evident in variations in intra-ethnic-group pain intensity. Within-group variation in reported pain intensity was most often associated with differences in degree of heritage consistency and LOC style. There was a significant interaction between ethnic identity and LOC style in the intragroup intensity analyses; specifically, the Anglo American and Polish groups demonstrated a different sort of relationship between pain-intensity variation and LOC style than did the other four groups (figure 4.2). Within these two groups, the subgroup with an internal style had a higher mean for pain intensity than the subgroup with an external style (in the Anglo American group the difference was significant—$F = 3.9$, $p < .05$—while in the Polish group it approached but did not attain statistical significance). Within each of the other four ethnic groups, by contrast, the subgroup with an internal style had a lower intensity mean than the subgroup with an external style (a difference of statistical significance only in the Latino group—$F = 5.01$, $p < .05$—and the French Canadian group—$F = 3.93$, $p < .05$). (Figure 4.3 illustrates the interaction of LOC style and ethnic identity in pain-intensity variation.)

In the five non–Anglo American groups, high heritage consistency was associated with lower pain intensities, although the association only attained statistical significance in the French Canadian and Irish groups (French Canadian group, $-.27$, $p = .05$; Irish group, $-.35$, $p = .02$).

With only one exception, there were no significant intragroup variations in reported pain intensity related to diagnosis, pain medications, religion, age, gender, workers' compensation status, or socioeconomic status (SES). The one exception was in the Irish group, which showed a significant difference in intensity related to occupation; the unskilled subgroup had the highest intensity mean of 44, while the skilled subgroup's mean of 26 was significantly lower ($F = 2.7$, $p < .05$).

In the total study population, there were also significant correlations between pain-intensity variation and the degrees of unhappiness, worry, fear, anger, tension, depression, and interference with work associated with the pain (table 4.1). In each response instance, as pain intensity

Figure 4.2. MPQ-PRIT by LOC Style in Ethnic Groups

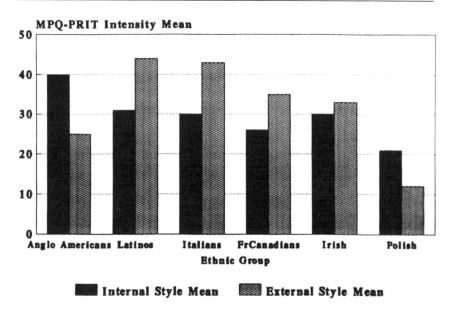

Figure 4.3. Pain Intensity by LOC Style by Ethnicity

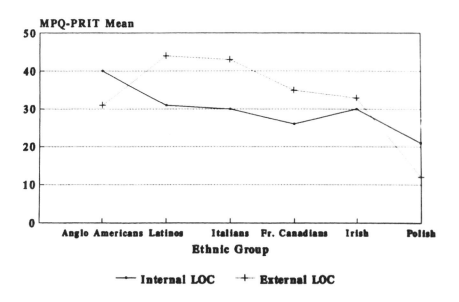

Table 4.1. Correlations between Total Pain Intensity (MPQ-PRIT) and Attitudinal, Behavioral, and Emotional/Psychological Responses

MPQ-PRIT and	Pearson Correlation Coefficients	p
Pain = Unhappiness	.26	.00
Degree of Anger	.20	.01
Degree of Expressiveness	.30	.00
Degree of Depression	.18	.01
Degree of Tension	.19	.01
Degree of Fear	.30	.00
Degree of Worries	.20	.00
Interference with Work	.18	.01

increased, the degree of behavioral impairment or emotional /psychological response increased as well.

Obviously, different culturally prescribed styles of describing pain may have affected patients' reports of pain severity. For example, it was clear that members of the Polish and Anglo American groups tended to be less expressive or emotional when describing their pain than were members of the Latino and Italian groups.

However, different reporting styles alone do not explain the correlations found between pain intensity and measures of behavioral and emotional response and life disruption (table 4.1). While pain intensity will of course affect pain response, it is also possible that the particular attitudes, beliefs, and cognitive styles associated with the different LOC styles and ethnic groups (to be discussed in detail in the next chapter) also influence pain perception.

This conclusion seems especially plausible given the absence of a statistically significant relationship in the pain center study between medical/biological factors and pain-intensity variation. And in other studies, evidence is mounting that learned cognitive influences, such as attitudes, meanings, and degree of attention to pain, may affect perceptions of pain severity (Wall and Melzack 1984, 1989; Maciewicz and Sandrew 1985; Chapman 1984; Fields and Basbaum 1989).

CASE STUDIES ILLUSTRATING CULTURAL
INFLUENCES ON REPORTED PAIN INTENSITY

Two case studies from the pain center study help to illustrate the cultural mediation of the chronic pain experience. The first case study demonstrates a familiar pattern among Latino men both in New England and in Puerto Rico. In his mid-thirties, Juan is a native of Puerto Rico who came to the U.S. mainland in the late 1970s. Juan is married and has three young children. Several other members of his family are also in New England and they all live in the same neighborhood; he socializes and interacts with them regularly. Juan came to the mainland because he believes strongly in the American dream. On numerous occasions he told me, "In America you can be anything you want to be." He believed that his move from Puerto Rico to the mainland would eventually lead to prosperity and an improved standard of living for himself and his family. He was very concerned that his children and future grandchildren have a better life than he had when living on the island.

Juan injured his back originally in the early 1980s while at work as a laborer, and had surgery involving the removal of a herniated disk in his lower back. He was able to return to work for two years, during which he was promoted to foreman, but in 1984 he reinjured his back on the job and since then has had chronic low-back pain and has been unable to return to work. He has not been considered a good candidate for repeat surgery. His diagnosis was postsurgical radicular low-back pain, which is pain caused by inflammation of the spinal nerve roots. Since the summer of 1986 he has received regular intravenous lidocaine treatments at the pain center. Juan reported high interference with sleep, sports, social activities, walking, and work.

Typical of the majority of Latinos at the pain center, Juan was very expressive about his pain. He displayed a lot of pain behavior, wincing, grimacing, and groaning more often than most of the non-Latino patients observed. On some occasions this expression led to misunderstandings with center nurses, many of whom are Anglo Americans: their own cultural values probably contributed to their view of Juan's behavior as inappropriate; especially, they indicated, for a man.

Juan described his pain as very severe, said he was very depressed, and defined himself as unhealthy and disabled. Juan's high LOC score indicated an external style, and he said that his pain presently controls his life. Juan has said on numerous occasions: "I'm not the man I used to be." Although he has been receiving workers' compensation, he is not happy with his situation, as he believes a "real man" must work. (Of course, his workers' compensation benefits are low and do not provide him with the resources to make a better life for himself and his family.) Juan maintains a belief that he will eventually be able to return to his job, and he refused the permanent settlement proposed by the workers' compensation system. He believes he will eventually be able to return to work with his former employer if he does not settle with workers' compensation.

He told me several times that within two to three years he will be well enough to return to his former position as foreman. Thus, one of Juan's coping strategies has been to deny that the pain and disability are permanent. This denial is understandable in light of his firm belief in his ability to make a better life for himself and his family through his migration to the mainland. In addition, he saw his earlier promotion to foreman (which occurred after his first surgery and subsequent return to work) as proof that he is capable of attaining his dream of economic prosperity, and thus he clings to the belief that he will eventually return to work and prosper.

Although at the time the pain center study ended Juan had been on workers' compensation for almost four consecutive years, he continued to refuse the repeated and persistent offers of workers' compensation for a settlement. The workers' compensation system made no effort to work with Juan in retraining for a new position with his old employer or a new employer. His workers' compensation insurer wanted Juan to accept a permanent cash settlement of his case so he would no longer receive weekly benefits—the goal of the workers' compensation system is clearly to maintain the workers' compensation insurance company's profits and to settle long-term-disability cases as cheaply and quickly as possible.

In addition to the failure of the workers' compensation system to assist Juan in his goal to work again, the pain center's "occupational therapy" program also failed to assist Juan with his job concerns. Occupational therapy (which is not available in Spanish) was available to Juan as he spoke English but was of no real assistance with his occupational concerns. Occupational therapy, as practiced at the pain center at the time of the study, involved teaching patients skills of daily home life such as eating, dressing, and doing household chores—often with the use of some mechanical device or brace (which of course were sold to them by the medical center). "Occupational therapy" was not aimed at helping patients with tasks of employment or retraining so they could engage in a new occupation. No counseling of this type was available at the center or through the workers' compensation insurer.

The most striking feature of Juan's response to his pain has been the effect of his disability on his self-image. For Juan and other Latino men in New England, as well as men in Puerto Rico such as Jesus described in chapter 1, pain and the accompanying inability to work symbolize a loss of manhood and self-esteem, since manhood is associated with being a good provider and protector of the family. Among Latinos on the island and on the mainland, the definition of maleness alludes to a man's ability to be a good provider and protector of his family and to his ability to control his destiny and be self-sufficient, and not merely to the more popular and often cited attitudes and behaviors of machismo (Sanchez-Ayendez 1984:243; Ramirez 1992).

Our next case study, Jane, offers a sharp contrast to Juan's chronic pain experience. Jane is a native of New England. She is a married woman who described herself as a New England "Yankee." A former nurse and now a full-time housewife in her late forties, she is from a lower middle-class background. She has several grown children and two very young grandchildren who live outside of New England. She said some of her greatest pleasures in life are the periodic visits her children and grandchildren make to visit her. Her husband is retired from military service and his pension is sufficient so that Jane does not have to work. Since her chronic pain makes nursing duties difficult, she ceased employment outside the home in the early 1980s, although she does sell some of her handmade crafts at local craft shows and fairs.

Jane has had chronic pain in her lower back and legs since the mid-1970s and has had disk surgery. She also has postsurgical radicular low-back pain and degenerative joint disease of the spine. In addition, she has arthritis and has had related surgeries on her knees and shoulders.

For most of her adult life, in addition to fulfilling her roles as wife and mother, Jane worked as a nurse at various hospitals in the United States. Her husband's military duties took the family to several different locations within the United States, and with each new move Jane found employment as a nurse. She continued to work for several years after her pain began. She said she did enjoy nursing, but the back pain and arthritis made it increasingly difficult to perform her duties. When her husband retired in the early 1980s, they returned permanently to New England, where Jane had been born and raised, and she decided to retire as well and became a full-time housewife.

Jane has been coming to the center since 1986. When first seen at the pain center, Jane was suffering from sleep disturbances related to the severity of her pain. At that time, she was also dependent on a prescription opiate analgesic for pain relief and was suffering from depression. She reports that the period just preceding her admission was one of the "bleakest" of her lifetime, she was unable to sleep or engage in meaningful social activities because the pain was so severe. She reported to me that she had become dependent on her opiate medications although they did not eliminate her chronic pain. Jane said she lost all sense of control over her life and her pain during this "bleak" period. Just prior to her first visit to the pain center, she was hospitalized at the medical center where the pain center is located for extreme exhaustion and depression. The attending physician for her inpatient stay referred her to the pain center upon her discharge.

Since coming to the pain center, Jane reported that her weekly treatments, which involve an infusion of intravenous lidocaine, provided about 60% pain relief, so that she now reports a low pain intensity level. At the time of the study she reported no depression and defined herself as healthy. She reported severe interference with sports and minor interference with walking.

Jane has taken a nonexpressive approach to living with her pain; she never displayed any pain behavior during interviews. She demonstrates a pattern found among many Anglo Americans. This pattern involves a lack of expressiveness and behavioral pain response, including very little wincing or groaning. This stoic behavior was highly approved of by the nurses at the center, who saw Jane as an ideal patient. Indeed, the Anglo American patients who behaved in this manner were welcomed by the nurses each week in a manner which showed respect and concern—a contrast to the judgmental and disapproving manner in which the expressive Latino or Italian patients were often treated.

Jane said she keeps very busy with crafts, sewing, reading, and visiting because activity keeps her mind off her pain, and she reported that when she was busy the pain seemed less severe. This tendency to "keep busy" as a coping strategy was found among numerous Anglo Americans and probably relates to the "Protestant work ethic" background of many members of this group (see Good 1992, Bellah et al. 1985, and Rubin 1976 for discussions of the value of work in Anglo American culture).

I saw Jane weekly during the study period and she was almost always cheerful and spoke of family visits and gatherings and craft fairs which she attended and which she clearly found very pleasurable. She often brought in samples of the crafts she made and sold at craft fairs so that the nurses and I could see them. She was clearly a person who found pleasure and fulfillment in her life despite her continued pain and arthritic and back problems.

Jane said she has some control over the pain through keeping busy and active and through her firm decision not to have further surgery (in her estimation her previous surgeries aggravated her pain). The strategies she employed to cope with and reduce her pain seemed to be fairly effective, and when I left the clinic at the end of the study Jane continued to do well by her own reports and those of her providers.

DISCUSSION

Although they both suffer from postsurgical radicular low-back pain, Juan and Jane differed not only in behavioral and psychological pain responses but also in the meanings they attached to their pain. For example, within the context of his culturally shaped definition of the male role, for Juan the chronic pain represented a loss of his manhood; but to Jane, a former nurse who accepted the biomedical model as a valid explanatory system, the pain signified a biological abnormality which she believed could be lived with and treated. Furthermore, Jane and Juan had different economic situations, which clearly affected the meanings they attached to their pain. Jane had access to sufficient economic resources from her husband's pension and had no personal-identity problems with ceasing employment outside the home; she was able to find personal satisfaction in craftmaking and social activities. In contrast, Juan had major economic problems and he clung to the economic dream he came to the mainland with—the dream of attaining a better life for his family. In Juan's view, responsibility for attainment of that dream rested on his shoulders as the man of the family, and he believed he was failing at that responsibility because of his chronic pain—thus, in addition to the strain of living in poverty, his personal identity was severely affected by his inability to work.

Although from a biomedical standpoint Jane's physical condition was considered more severe than Juan's, Juan perceived more severe pain and life disruption and expressed more negative responses to the pain. This research suggests that this is in part due to the different meanings he attached to his pain. In order to understand why Juan was experiencing more severe pain than Jane, we must expand our vision beyond the traditional biomedical model based on mind-body dualism. Those who insist on strict adherence to the mind-body dualism concept will insist that Juan's pain was not really more severe—that he simply was more expressive—because by biomedical standards he had less bodily damage than Jane. This view disregards the reality of Juan's pain experience. Weekly or biweekly visits with both Juan and Jane made it very clear that Juan was suffering more severe pain and certainly experiencing more severe life disruption and depression than Jane.

Qualitative data from this pain center study suggest that different reporting styles alone do not entirely explain why the Latinos and Italians reported higher pain intensities than, for example, the Anglo American and Polish patients. The evidence suggests that members of certain ethnic groups (and members of the external LOC-style group) did experience more severe pain as well as more severe life disruptions.

A BIOCULTURAL MODEL OF PAIN PERCEPTION

In order to conceptualize how culturally shaped attitudes and meanings can affect perceptions of pain intensity, I proposed that a biocultural model may provide an appropriate heuristic basis for illustrating the complex relationship between cultural influences and pain perception (Bates 1987; Bates et al. 1993) (see figure 4.4). This model integrates aspects of gate-control theory (Melzack and Wall 1965; Wall and Melzack 1984, 1989) with social learning and social comparison theories (Bandura 1977). Figure 4.4 suggests that the source of social comparison is home and family, where adults transmit to children the values and attitudes of their cultural or ethnic group. Attitudes, expectations, meanings for experiences, and appropriate emotional expressiveness are learned through observing the reactions and behaviors of others who are similar in identity to oneself. The pain center study found ethnic differences in accepted standards for and attitudes toward pain and pain behavior within defined ethnic groups.

The biocultural model of pain perception does not assume any basic differences in the neurophysiology of members of different ethnic groups. People learn in social communities, where conventional ways of interpreting, expressing, and responding to pain are acquired. People with similar learning experiences are likely to show similar pain perception, expression, and response patterns. This patterning of pain perception and response is cultural and, as such, may influence the neurophysiological processing of nociceptive information as well as psychological, behavioral, and verbal responses to pain. These effects on the pain experience may occur through various supraspinal influences on pain perception that were discussed in chapter 2, and which also are detailed in Wall and Melzack (1989) and Fields and Basbaum (1989).

Although it is likely that intense pain can affect attention, attitudes, and emotions, it is also possible that attitudes, degree of attention, and emotions were influencing perceptions of pain intensity in the pain center study population. In addition, different culturally prescribed styles of describing the pain may have affected the patients' reports of pain severity. As noted, members of the Polish and Anglo American groups tended to be less expressive or emotional when describing their pain than were members of the Latino and Italian groups. These differences appeared in both the ethnographic data and the affective category of the MPQ, where the Latino and Italian groups had the highest and second-highest means respectively. However, different reporting styles alone do not seem to explain the correlations between pain intensity reports and measures of response such as work stoppage and other forms of life disruption to be presented in the next chapter. In addition, cognitive influences, such as attitudes and degree of attention to pain, may affect perceptions of pain severity. Therefore, if one is raised in a cultural environment which defines focusing one's attention on the pain as either an appropriate or

Figure 4.4. Biocultural Model of Pain Perception

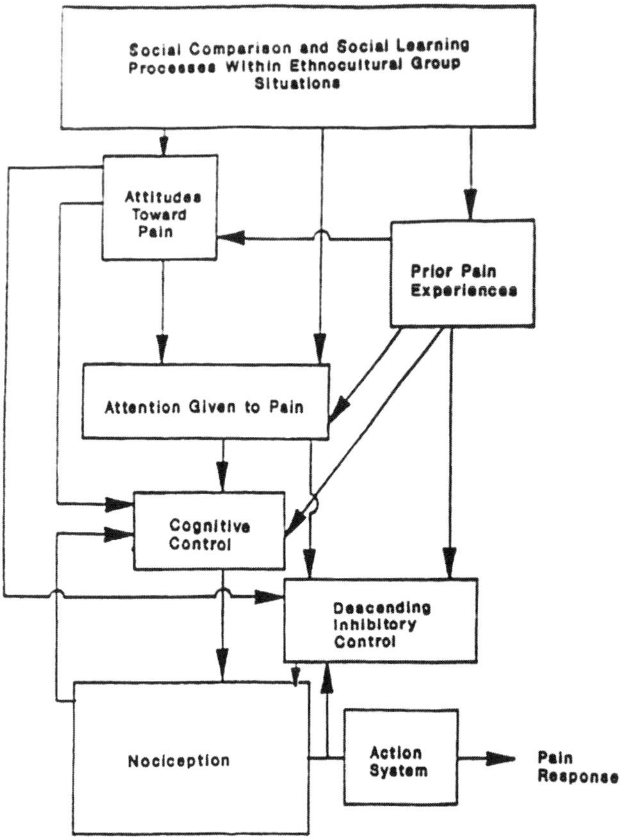

inappropriate response, this culturally acquired pattern may not only lead to certain styles of reporting but also may affect the actual perception of the pain.

The IASP taxonomy notes: "Pain is always subjective. Each individual learns the application of the word through experiences related to injury in early life. It is unquestionably a sensation in a part of the body but it is also always unpleasant and therefore also an emotional experience" (Merskey 1979). This holds true for several of the groups at the pain center, for whom cultural background was significantly related to differences in reported perception of total pain intensity described in both sensory and affective terms.

The next chapter offers an in-depth discussion, including quantitative analyses and materials from case studies, which further illustrate ethnic differences in pain reporting and responses.

CHAPTER 5

INTER- AND INTRA-ETHNIC-GROUP VARIATIONS IN PAIN RESPONSES IN THE NEW ENGLAND POPULATION

Despite the claims of many specialists in the chronic pain field that most chronic pain patients are very much alike, and that the vast majority experience the same "chronic pain career"—as well as the obvious stereotyping of these patients in the existing literature (Aronoff 1985, Kotarba 1983, Lindsay and Wyckoff 1981)—the New England study found substantial differences in the chronic pain experiences of the center's patients. Case studies from the New England study demonstrate that while some patients have experienced high degrees of pain intensity, depression, anger, worry, tension, and unhappiness, others have adapted quite well to their pain experiences and found ways to adjust their behavior and attitudes to lead lives, defined by the participants, as productive, happy, and worthwhile.

QUALITATIVE FINDINGS OF PAIN RESPONSE VARIATION

All qualitative data were coded and analyzed regarding stages in the chronic pain experience, including the initial injury or illness episode; subsequent diagnostic, treatment, and surgical events; remission periods, if any; encounters with providers defined by patients as helpful or unhelpful; family and work problems or changes; and present status. The content analyses also involved the search for and coding of consistent themes and key words or phrases.

The pain experiences revealed by members of four of the New England ethnic groups illustrate diverse responses to the chronic pain both between and within ethnic groups.

The Anglo American Chronic Pain Experience

Among Anglo Americans, a theme that emerged from the qualitative data was one of "working and keeping busy" to take their minds off their pain. This coping strategy is probably related to the "Protestant work ethic" background of many Anglo Americans. Tropman (1989:98, 131–132) and Good (1992:50–51) recently discussed and demonstrated the continuing importance and dominance of the American cultural value of work and the continuing influence of the "Protestant work ethic" in contemporary Anglo-American culture.

A second trend at the New England pain center was a lack of expressiveness and behavioral pain response among most Anglo Americans (i.e., stoicism), including very little wincing or groaning. Good (1992:64) also found stoicism to be associated with pain behavior of some Anglo Americans in her study. This stoic behavior was highly valued by the New England center's nursing staff, many of whom shared a similar cultural background with this group. Indeed, the Anglo American patients who behaved in this manner were treated with respect and approval by the nurses, in contrast to the disapproval often shown to the expressive Latino and Italian patients.

Jane, the case study in chapter 4, was one such Anglo American who demonstrated this tendency to be nonexpressive about pain. Jane was very stoic and never displayed any pain behavior in my presence. Nurses at the center saw Jane as an ideal patient.

Jane also demonstrated another trend evident in the Anglo American group—the general acceptance of the biomedical worldview of the body as a machine-like entity separate from the mind. To Jane, her pain signified a biological abnormality that could be treated and lived with. In her case, biomedical treatment at the center was proving to be of some value in reducing (but not eliminating) the pain.

Despite Jane's rather positive case study and her good relationships with the providers at the center, the congruence between the worldviews of health-care providers and Anglo American patients did not always lead to a satisfactory relationship between them. Because many Anglo Americans have accepted the legitimacy and effectiveness of biomedicine, if such treatment proved ineffective, members of this group often became extremely angry at individual providers when they were unable to effectively repair the body and free it of pain. However, this anger did not for the most part lead to abandoning biomedicine in general, but rather to continuing the quest for the one biomedical physician who would finally find and fix the mechanical problem the patient believed must be causing his or her pain.

One extreme example of this quest involved an Anglo American, Mary, who has had chronic pain since the early 1980s. Mary, a large woman in her fifties who speaks very loudly, keeps her body constantly in motion, waving her arms violently and often. She has an eighth-grade education and was a former nurse's aide, but at the time of the study was unemployed and receiving Social Security disability benefits. The mother of three grown children, Mary was not married at the time of the study.

According to her medical record, Mary suffers from arthritis, fibromyalgia, low-back pain, chronic musculoskeletal pain syndrome, carpal tunnel syndrome, depression, and severe sleep disturbances. She has a medical history of cardiac problems and had related triple coronary-bypass surgery in 1983. She also has had several disks removed, several shoulder surgeries, a hysterectomy, breast surgery for a cyst, hemorrhoid surgery, various foot operations (for torn ligaments), hernia repair, numerous D and Cs, a spinal fusion, and multiple other surgeries. At the time of the study she was taking numerous medications for her cardiac problems, antidepressants, and several nonopiate pain medications. Mary completed the stress-reduction program at the New England center with a perfect attendance record, but the doctors reported that it had little impact on her symptoms or life style.

According to the medical record, Mary also has a long history of depression, suicidal gestures, and hospitalization for psychiatric problems in various state mental hospitals. She has a history of receiving psychotropic medications but was not receiving psychiatric treatment when she first sought care at the New England center in 1984. After her initial evaluation at the New England center, it was decided that she should have further outpatient treatment for depression, should take an antidepressant medication, and should receive weekly intravenous lidocaine infusions at the New England center to reduce her pain intensity. She was still receiving the infusions throughout the study, during which I saw her weekly or biweekly.

Unlike many Anglo Americans, Mary was expressive about her pain. Week after week she complained loudly of the severity of her pain to me and to other patients (patients receiving intravenous lidocaine infusions were in a large treatment room together, and each procedure took from one to three hours to complete). Each time I saw Mary she claimed to be much worse than the last time we met. Each week, when asked by nurses to rank her pain on a 0 to 10 scale, she always reported a 10. When I visited with other patients in the I.V. procedure room, Mary often sought my attention and loudly demanded to be heard over others.

When first interviewed, Mary said her pain became chronic after 1983 bypass surgery. She said she experienced severe pain everywhere and on numerous occasions asserted that the physicians were not giving her enough pain medication. When I suggested that this was because the doctors did not want her to become addicted to the medications, she said, "Oh, I never abuse it." On that occasion, she had her daughter with her and the daughter caught my eye and shook her head to indicate that Mary was not being truthful about her medication use (her daughter thought Mary did engage in medication abuse).

Mary, who lives in the same neighborhood as two of her children and several siblings (she is one of ten children), nieces, and nephews, interacts regularly with her extended family. According to Mary, some of her relatives have been supportive while others have contributed to substantial stress in her life. She frequently talked at length about her family and family problems, and during the study she reported that two of her sisters had died. She also talked at length about her boyfriend of seven years, whom she became engaged to during the research period.

Over the months that I visited with Mary, it became clear that she did not understand the nature of her condition—although physicians did attempt explanations. The medical record indicates the physicians recognized Mary's difficulty with comprehension and, according to notes in her record, her New England center attending physician's view was that she has "difficulty with abstract reasoning." Other medical notes from a neurological consult requested by the New England center physician indicate that tests revealed Mary was "functioning well below average in the borderline range of intelligence. She shows some capacity for memory encoding, but generally shows below average functioning across a variety of tasks that were assessed." The evaluation indicates it could not be determined if this was, at least in part, due to emotional distress or other causes. (At that time her I.Q. tested in the 77 to 78 range; however, her memory function test scores were higher than her intellectual scores.) The same report recommended further psychotherapeutic intervention.

For whatever reasons, Mary did not comprehend the nature or causes of her emotional and physical conditions and said that her pain comes from "a wire they put in my chest when they operated on my heart. It's to hold my rib cage together."

When I saw Mary during 1987 and 1988, she had already had thirty-three operations, none of which she felt helped reduce her pain level. She was planning to have further surgery when the study concluded. She blamed individual surgeons for personal incompetence, but even after thirty-three operations she still believed there was a cure.

There were several factors in Mary's history, including a lack of education beyond eighth grade (which probably in part explains why she did not seem to understand her conditions), the recent deaths and associated loss of several close relatives, and a lack of confidence due to past failed personal relationships, that contributed to Mary's sense of not having control over her life. The perceived lack of control along with her inability to comprehend the nature of her medical and psychological problems have rendered Mary unable to question surgeries proposed by the many doctors she has consulted.

Mary's overall locus-of-control (LOC) scores indicated a strong external style. She does not believe she possesses the ability to overcome her pain and instead continues to search for the one surgeon who can "fix" it. Despite the failure of thirty-three surgeries to free her of pain, Mary still did not question the ultimate legitimacy of biomedicine. She steadfastly maintained that a competent surgeon would relieve her pain in her upcoming thirty-fourth surgery!

Many other Anglo Americans were angered by the suggestion that their pain problem had any psychological component. Given their acceptance of the mind-body dualism concept, they believed the pain was either biological or mental and that their own pain was definitely biological in nature. Any suggestion that psychological components might aggravate or be related to the pain made them angry because they interpreted this to mean that "the doctor thinks it's all in my head."

This was not an unrealistic interpretation, as the doctors at this so-called multidisciplinary clinic did appear to prefer biomedical interventions (such as nerve blocks, epidural steroid injections, and intravenous medications) wherever possible. Although the initial evaluation of each patient included a psychological evaluation, the major focus was on the biological aspects of, and biological treatments for, the pain. Despite physicians' claims of believing in a biopsychosocial model of chronic pain treatment, there remained much evidence of the mind-body dualism concept present in actual clinical practice. Most patients were first treated for biological abnormalities or symptoms using biomedical methods, and only if those proved ineffective through time or if patients clearly exhibited severe psychological stress (such as threats of suicide) did physicians focus on psychosocial aspects of the chronic pain and refer patients for psychological treatments.

Joe is one Anglo American male subject who expressed displeasure with suggestions for psychological counseling which were offered by New England center physicians after biomedical treatment had been tried for some time. Joe, a native of New England, has suffered from postsurgical low-back pain and was recently diagnosed as also having degenerative disk disease. A married man with two teenage children, Joe earned a high school education. In his late forties when interviewed in 1987 and

1988, he had had back pain for more than four years and, in 1987, had been coming to the New England center for about nine months.

Joe was not considered a candidate for repeat back surgery. He was receiving periodic epidural steroid injections and oral anti-inflammatory medications for his back problems at the New England center but still reported significant levels of pain and associated depression and anger. After several months of no significant long-term improvement from physical therapy and the steroid injections, he somewhat reluctantly participated in the New England center's stress reduction course. However, he refused to follow his New England center physician's most recent advice to see the center psychologist on a regular basis, explaining that "My pain is in my back, not in my head."

Joe originally injured his back while working as a tradesman for a construction company. At that time, Joe had disk surgery and returned to work for eighteen months following his surgical recovery. After the initial injury, Joe received medical and wage compensation benefits from workers' compensation. However, when he began experiencing back problems eighteen months after his surgery, his workers' compensation insurer initially denied his claim, saying his current back problems were not attributable to his earlier on-the-job injury.

Joe did not express his pain behaviorally—there was no wincing or groaning. However, he was angry about the way his case had been handled by his workers' compensation insurer. Joe described how devastated he felt when he had to stop working the second time and workers' compensation denied his second claim. While appealing to the state workers' compensation board, a process which took almost two years, he had no income or health insurance. (As Joe's condition was not defined as a permanent disability, he was not eligible for Social Security Disability Insurance [SSDI] benefits.) Unable to pay rent during that time, Joe and his family lost their apartment and had to move in with Joe's parents, who lived in the area. After several months, Joe's wife (previously a full-time housewife and mother) found work as a waitress, although her income made the family ineligible for Medicaid; her job offered no health insurance. Despite her income, the family was not able to secure housing of its own until the workers' compensation board finally ruled in Joe's favor two years after the second claim was originally denied.

During this appeals process, Joe became very fearful of engaging in any physical activity and, as he had no health insurance, he did not receive occupational therapy or rehabilitation services during that two year period. He believed, he told us, that workers' compensation agents rode through neighborhoods trying to find compensation claimants engaging in physical tasks that would prove the workers did not deserve benefits. As a result of the adversarial relationship between Joe and his workers' compensation insurer, his fears were very real and led to a very inactive and unhappy existence for him. Without that fearful two-year period, he might have become involved in rehabilitative activities that might have reduced some of his back pain and associated disability.

When first interviewed in 1987, Joe had been receiving workers' compensation benefits for about ten months following his successful appeal; however, the previous two-year appeal period had instilled in him a not-unreasonable fear of engaging in even those household, yard, and recreational activities he was capable of performing. As a result of his fears, he reported severe interference in all daily activities and believed that his life would remain unhappy as long as he had any degree of back pain. The only way to continue to have an income and health benefits, he felt, was to remain on workers' compensation—any trial attempt on his part to return to some type of work might ultimately fail and result in the loss of this security. Thus, he clung to his hard-won workers' compensation benefits as his only hope of avoiding complete financial disaster of the kind he had recently experienced. At the end of the New England study, Joe remained an unhappy man who reported substantial anger at the workers' compensation system which, in his view, trapped him in a system that provided little hope of real rehabilitation.

The Latino Chronic Pain Experience

Among all six New England ethnic groups, the Latino group, made up mainly of Puerto Rican immigrants to the mainland, was the most recent group to arrive in the United States. Many island Puerto Ricans migrate to the mainland, permanently or temporarily, for economic reasons that often are associated with unemployment and a surplus of labor on the island related to economic transformations which yielded many displaced and surplus workers (Reyes and Inclan 1991:1; Rodriguez 1991:6; Morales 1986).

As noted in chapter 4, the majority of Latinos were born outside the U.S. mainland, and the Latino group had the highest mean score for heritage consistency—indicating strong ties to the local ethnic community and a lifestyle reflective of the group's ethnic heritage. It has been noted that among U.S. mainland immigrant Puerto Ricans, maintenance of a self-identification as Puerto Rican is common. Even among Puerto Ricans born on the mainland, self-identification as Puerto Rican, or as bicultural, rather than total assimilation to an American identity, is reported (Rodriguez 1991).

Certainly, migration to the mainland is associated with cultural changes and a certain degree of acculturation, and reports of generational conflict regarding values has been noted in the literature (Ghali 1977, 1982; Szalay and Diaz-Guerrero 1985; Schensul, Nieves, and Martinez 1982, Canino and Canino 1980; Rogler, Cortez, and Malgady 1991). Nonetheless, many researchers studying Puerto Ricans living on the mainland report a continued self-identification as Puerto Rican, a continued reliance on certain Puerto Rican cultural values and traditional forms of social support, and a continued use of Spanish at home as a "marker of cultural, social, and political identity" (Duran 1983:27, Sanchez-Ayendez 1988, Rodriguez 1991:17).

Rodriguez notes that external factors also contribute to continuation of Puerto Rican ethnic identity and to the incidence of biculturalism rather than total acculturation among mainland Puerto Ricans: "The long-lasting quality of Puerto Rican identity is also related to the disadvantaged position of the group as a whole. . . . Residential segregation or concentration has also had an impact on the ethnic identification of Puerto Ricans . . . [including] the concentration of Hispanic children in particular schools" (1991:18). Tienda also notes that this sustained Puerto Rican identity is due to the "continued revitalization of ethnic symbols through the process of labor migration [constant back-and-forth migration from island to mainland]" (1985). This back-and-forth migration is, of course, related to external factors such as colonization of the island and associated economic conditions. Although not all Puerto Ricans are involved in this back-and-forth migration, "for an individual to function in both or either community, in familial networks, and the general community, it is important that he or she be both bilingual and bicultural" (Rodriguez 1991:18).

Many of the Puerto Rican immigrants in the New England study lived among other Puerto Ricans, including extended family members, and had very strong ties to the local Latino community. Almost universally these participants reported high degrees of family interdependence. Many also reported periodic trips back to the island to visit family and friends. All Puerto Ricans interviewed in New England self-identified as Puerto Rican rather than as Americans.

One theme which emerged among Latino men in New England was their sense of having lost their manhood if they could no longer work. While numerous men from all six groups expressed worries related to ceasing employment, this situation had a greater effect on the self-image of Latino men. For them, chronic pain symbolized a loss of manhood because the pain was associated with a self-perceived inability to be a good provider and protector of the family. As noted in chapter 4, this attitude seems understandable given the cultural outlook on manhood held by this ethnic group.

Numerous men in the Latino group reported a great loss of self-esteem, which resulted in associated depression. Similar to Juan's case (see chapter 4) was that of Ricardo, another Latino man who had postsurgical radicular low-back pain following three surgeries to remove herniated disks. Ricardo, in his mid-thirties, had been in pain for seven years and had been coming to the New England center for over three years when I met him in 1987.

A former semiskilled laborer with a high school education, Ricardo came to the mainland from Puerto Rico about ten years ago, believing that here he could build a better life for himself and his family. The back pain forced him to cease work, and initially he was denied workers' compensation benefits—at that time his wife had to find a job and became the sole supporter of the family. Eventually, his workers' compensation appeal did result in benefits being awarded; however, his workers' compensation weekly checks were only $140.00, so his wife has had to continue to work outside the home. Ricardo was greatly distressed about his inability to work and about his wife's new role.

His wife, who accompanied him to the clinic, said, "He really likes to work. He says 'now you're the man and I'm like the woman.'" Ricardo was very upset that his wife, who used to stay at home, now must work to help support the family. In addition, his back pain is so severe that his wife has had to do all of the driving, including bringing him in for his pain center visits, all of which also disturbs Ricardo. Overall, as with Juan, his sense of manhood has been negatively affected by his pain and inability to work. His anger and frustration were clearly affecting his relationship with his wife, who said Ricardo gets very impatient and "yells" at her when the pain gets bad.

The inability (or unwillingness) of both the workers' compensation system and the New England center's occupational therapy program to assist Ricardo with his occupational concerns was clearly one major factor in his anger and frustration. Ricardo wanted desperately to work again, yet no one at the workers' compensation insurance company or in the center's occupational therapy program was assisting him in retraining for a nonmanual occupation. Ricardo has a high school education and he spoke English well. Given these advantages, it did not seem unrealistic to imagine that there was some type of work that he could be retrained to do. However, the current medical and compensation systems of the United States generally are not structured to work with individuals in making and carrying out plans for retraining. In addition, Ricardo's workers' compensation benefits were so low that no money was available for

Ricardo to finance his own retraining or pursue higher education. Under such an ineffective system, it is not surprising that Ricardo was angry and frustrated, especially since he believed his entire manhood was adversely affected by his inability to work and be a good provider for his family.

A second theme in the Latino group was a marked tendency on the part of both men and women to express pain verbally and behaviorally (wincing, groaning, grimacing) much more often than did members of the Anglo American and Polish groups. Even among Latinos who were adjusting to their pain experiences quite effectively and who thought they had a happy and fulfilled life despite the pain, expressiveness of pain was quite high. This expressiveness often led to problems with the New England center nursing staff, many of whom said they believed this expressiveness to be inappropriate—especially in men. About Juan, one nurse said, "He starts to yell when I apply the alcohol swab—even before I put in the needle [for the I.V.]. He looks so macho but he acts like a baby." Clearly, different cultural beliefs about acceptable behavior have led to problems in the patient-nurse relationship at the New England center.

Yolanda, a Puerto Rican immigrant to the mainland, also illustrates this Latino trend toward expressiveness. Yolanda, in her mid-thirties, had one year of nurse's aide education beyond high school and worked as a nurse's aide at a New England nursing home before her pain began. She said she injured her back in an accident on the job but she did not receive workers' compensation for the injury.

According to her physicians, Yolanda suffers from mechanical and radicular low-back pain with some evidence of degenerative joint disease of the spine. She had been in chronic pain for six months when I first interviewed her. Yolanda has not had any back surgeries and takes anti-inflammatories and antidepressants for her pain. Despite the medications, the pain has made it difficult for her to do her housework, to walk for any distance, and to sit for long periods. She has not been able to return to her job and reported high interference with her normal work of household chores and child care. She has found it increasingly difficult to care for her eight-month-old baby and six-year-old son and said the pain is affecting her marriage, including her sexual relations. She reported moaning and groaning and crying frequently in response to her pain.

Yolanda used a TENS unit (see Glossary) for pain relief but did not like to do so. She said, "I feel like my life is being run by a machine—at times I feel like a robot. I get very depressed because of the pain but there is not much I could do to avoid the pain from coming back."

She reported that the pain has affected her social life with old friends, which she said was very active before the pain. She also was concerned that she could no longer help her friends and relatives. She said, "I used to do so much for others and now I can't. This gets me very depressed and sad." Yolanda appeared to be more stressed about her failure to fulfill social roles than about having to cease employment.

Yolanda expressed anger that no one has been able to really help her get rid of the pain and she blamed the nursing home for her injury and for not providing her with workers' compensation after the accident. No one at the New England center made any effort to assist Yolanda with appealing the workers' compensation insurer's denial of benefits or to help her retrain for a new position. Yolanda did not have sufficient funds to hire a lawyer to represent her in a court appeal of the workers' compensation decision. Thus, as with Ricardo, the New England center's occupational therapy program as well as the workers' compensation system were providing no assistance to Yolanda. She was not even receiving minimal workers' compensation benefits, even though she said she was injured on the job. Yolanda's case was not unique. Many patients from all ethnic groups reported problems with the workers' compensation system— some of these problems were discussed earlier in this chapter.

No one at the pain center assisted Yolanda in trying to obtain compensation from her former employer, nor did they assist her with her depression. Although Yolanda did speak some English, she was not fluent enough to take the psychological tests that are generally part of the admission packet, and thus received neither psychological assessment nor psychological treatments. This was not uncommon at the center, since there was no translator available for Spanish speaking patients and none of the admission questionnaires and psychological tests were available in Spanish. (The MPQ also was not available in Spanish until I brought it to the New England center during the study and administered it to all Spanish-speaking patients during the research period.) As a result of the unavailability of services in Spanish, Yolanda received no help with her psychosocial needs; instead, the pain center's staff focused on her biological symptoms, providing prescriptions for medications and a TENS unit.

Indeed, Yolanda was more fortunate than most Latinos at the center—she could speak enough English to communicate her condition to the physicians. Many other Latinos who spoke only Spanish brought an 8-to-10-year-old boy or girl (a child or grandchild) to the clinic to translate their concerns to physicians. Understandably, such translations often led to miscommunications between providers and patients. When I discussed this situation with the director of the pain center, he was very concerned, even though state and institutional budget problems prohibited him from hiring a translator for the Latino patients. (The budget problems at the medical center, related to the larger political and economic conditions in the state at the time, also led to a reduction in both physicians and nurses at the pain center during my research—while at the same time the administration of the medical center wanted the pain center's patient load to be increased, all of which led to ever-increasing stress on providers and patients.)

Yolanda reported that she feels she has little or no control over the direction her life is taking and feels as if the pain controls her life much of the time. She was very expressive about her pain, anger, depression, and frustration, and at our last interview said, "I used to be a very active woman, now I always ache. I now live in Hell town."

Yolanda's open expressions of pain intensity, depression, anger, and frustration made her unpopular with the center's nursing staff because she did not meet their expectations for appropriate behavior. As a result, the pain center was not a supportive environment for Yolanda.

While Latino expressiveness in New England led to patient-provider relationship problems, the research I have been conducting on the island of Puerto Rico has revealed that island health-care providers view patients' expressiveness as appropriate, and thus patients in Puerto Rico meet no discrimination or disapproval from island health-care providers. However, expressive Latino (and Italian) patients in New England often met with provider disapproval.

It is clear from my current project in Puerto Rico (discussed in detail in the next chapter) that the cultural context of medical care is very different on the island. Since the majority of Latino patients in New England were immigrants from the island, they have clearly experienced difficulties at the pain center in part because the cultural context of medical care has been so different in New England compared to the health-care system on their native island. In addition, of course, the Latinos at the pain center often encountered the language barrier and associated communication problems discussed earlier.

The Polish Chronic Pain Experience

Two Polish case studies demonstrate a very different culturally shaped pattern of response to the chronic pain experience than what was found among the New England Latinos.

Carl is a second-generation Polish American who is now in his early thirties. He reported strong ties to the local Polish American community and was close to his extended family. He also reported that during his lifetime he has experienced some discrimination because he is Polish, but still feels pride in being a "Polish American." He has an associate's degree and worked as a professional before his accident.

Carl is married but as yet has no children. He said his medical problems have not adversely affected his marriage, but he did report difficulty with sexual relations due to the pain. Despite this difficulty, Carl continually told me the pain had not affected his relationship with his wife. Given that he was only in his early thirties, his lack of expressed concern about the pain's effect on his sex life was somewhat surprising. Perhaps the Polish Americans' tendency to be stoic and nonexpressive about pain contributed to Carl's insistence that all was well in his marriage despite the difficulty with sexual relations.

Carl suffers from neck pain, radicular low-back with associated leg pain, and migraine headaches, which all began after he was in a motorcycle accident in 1985. At the time of the accident he underwent back surgery for a herniated disk. Before coming to the pain center he had been seen for his accident-related problems by a variety of doctors, including neurologists, neurosurgeons, a chiropractor, an osteopath, and a psychologist. Since coming to the pain center, he takes anti-inflammatories and opiate analgesics, and also is taking methadone in an attempt to lessen his use of opiates.

He has been unable to work due to his injuries, has been receiving Social Security disability benefits, and is in the process of litigation concerning the accident which caused his injuries (in his view, the driver of the car he collided with was at fault). In addition to his inability to work, Carl reported severe interference in social activities, household chores, sports, sleep, and sexual relations. His MPQ overall pain intensity score was 41, one of the highest scores in the Polish group, which had a MPQ mean of 29.2—the lowest of all ethnic groups.

Despite his high pain intensity score on the MPQ, Carl was very nonexpressive about his pain; he said he does not like to talk about the pain with others. He never displayed any pain behavior in my presence—this was common among the Polish, who tended to be as nonexpressive and stoic as many of the Anglo Americans. I often hesitate to describe these findings because I realize they confirm certain stereotypes; however, both the quantitative and qualitative data clearly show a strong tendency for nonexpressiveness among the Polish and the Anglo Americans and for expressiveness among Latinos and Italians—although as noted earlier, there was within-group variation in most response areas, including expressiveness.

Carl reported that, in his estimation, he is coping quite well with his pain and disability. He said two of his major coping strategies are to ignore the pain and to hide it from others. Another major strategy he has been employing is to return to school to study a craft he could engage in despite his pain. His studies keep him busy, he enjoys them, and he is preparing for a career to pursue despite his pain. Thus, Carl's substantial use of coping strategies has allowed him to live a life he defined as worthwhile. Carl strongly disagreed with the statement: "As long as I have pain I will never have a fulfilling and happy life."

Carl was very pleased to be on methadone because he wants to discontinue all opiate medications as soon as possible, although as yet he is unable to stand the pain without the methadone and the increasingly smaller doses of opiates. At the time the study concluded, Carl was coming to the pain center only for his methadone and Percocet prescriptions (which he was still decreasing) and was no longer receiving any other treatments. He was still in school and still defined himself as "healthy, but the pain has slowed me down."

It was clearly important to Carl to be viewed by others as healthy and normal, and he stressed numerous times his ability to hide his pain from others, saying "I'm an expert at it [hiding the pain]." Repeatedly stressing a belief in his ability to overcome the pain and medical problems, Carl said he was not depressed and his psychological evaluation by the pain center psychologist concurred. Overall, Carl appeared to be coping fairly well, employing coping mechanisms which were useful to him. Of course, if he is ultimately unsuccessful in discontinuing opiate medications, his use of opiates as a coping strategy may be a long-term disadvantage and maladaptive in the long run.

Wilma, in her mid-seventies, is a first generation Polish American. Despite their age difference, Wilma's response to pain and illness has been very similar to Carl's. Wilma suffers from chronic neck pain, chronic myofascial syndrome, and recurrent occipital neuralgia—all of which she said began when she was in an auto accident in 1986. Since she is suing the driver of the other automobile, she was at first reluctant to talk with me because of the litigation. But assured that her real name would not be used and that her research questionnaires would not be made available to anyone, including the other driver's insurance company, she agreed to participate.

Wilma's parents were both born in Poland, and Polish was the language spoken in her childhood home. As an adult, Wilma is fluent in English and also still speaks Polish. She is married, with six adult children. She reported strong ties to them, her grandchildren, her sibling, and the local Polish community. Retired since 1983 from a semiskilled factory job, Wilma enjoys walking, reading, and crocheting. However, she reported that her pain causes severe interference with sleep, social activities, driving, walking, and sexual relations. When she first came to the pain center, Wilma had a score of 55 on the MPQ—the highest score within the Polish group.

Like Carl, despite her high pain intensity, Wilma reported no depression. She also disagreed strongly with the statement linking pain with unhappiness and considered herself generally healthy with a slight disability only in regard to driving and heavy lifting. Despite the interference of pain with her daily activities, Wilma believed she was getting better and reported that her close family members have been very helpful and supportive.

She said, however, that since she does not like to discuss her pain, many of her friends do not even know she has the pain and medical problems. She said when the pain is bad she stays at home and does not communicate with her friends. She displayed no pain behavior at any time during the interviews.

One negative coping response (in Wilma's estimation) is that she "overeats" in response to her pain. She said as a result she is now very fat, although she looked very thin and her medical record indicated she had only gained three pounds. Nonetheless, her eating "problem" was a concern to Wilma. In addition, pending litigation against the other driver worried Wilma, and the uncertainty of its outcome was constantly on her mind. When I saw Wilma, this case had already been in process for almost two years and was not likely to be resolved for at least another year or two—this time frame appeared to be very common among patients involved in such cases. The lengthy litigation process due to delays in hearing cases in the state court system often contributed to substantial stress in the lives of the chronic pain patients at the pain center.

Wilma reported that prior to coming to the pain center, she worried a great deal that she had a brain tumor and that the pain would never decrease. However, she reported that treatment at the pain center (which included prescription anti-inflammatories, trigger point injections, and physical therapy) provided relief, and also the pain center physician's explanation of her pain has relieved her mind, so she no longer believes she has a brain tumor and feels reassured now about her physical condition.

As noted earlier, Carl's and Wilma's nonexpressive approach to pain was shared by most of the Polish Americans in this study. Their belief that pain does not have to lead to unhappy and unfulfilled lives was also shared by other Polish Americans; the Polish group had the lowest unhappiness mean of all six groups. In contrast to the Latino patients, and in part because of shared values about appropriate pain behavior, the Polish patients often had a good relationship with the pain center nurses and physicians. Many Polish patients, including Wilma and Carl, viewed the pain center as a supportive and helpful environment.

The Irish Chronic Pain Experience

Our first Irish case study, Betty, is 39 years of age. Her pain began in 1983, after cancer surgery and follow-up radiation therapy. She has had chronic pain ever since. She also has serious arthritic changes in numerous joints and has had multiple bone fractures related to the surgery and radiation. She was referred to the pain center in late 1984.

In her initial assessment, Betty was described by the center psychologist as a pleasant, verbal, friendly, and cooperative thirty-seven-year-old female. He noted that she described her illness and her attempts to deal with it clearly and that her optimistic, constructive outlook toward dealing with a serious illness was evident. He stated that she was obviously an individual who sought mastery over the difficulties that life had set before her and worked very hard to that end.

At the time of the study, Betty had very little depression associated with her pain. She reported the greatest degree of interference with walking, sports, and her former employment as a nurse. She still enjoyed social activities and told me her friendships have not been affected by her pain and medical problems.

During her initial treatment period at the center, Betty took opiate analgesics for several months; during the past two years, after she began receiving regular intravenous lidocaine infusions at the pain center, the pain relief she obtains from the infusions has allowed her to get off opiate medications. Now she takes antidepressants. She participated in the center's stress reduction and biofeedback program and reported that both were very helpful in reducing her pain. She regularly practiced visualization and meditation and found them useful. However, Betty still experienced some fairly severe pain at times which, when at its worst, she described as searing and stabbing.

Betty is a very positive person, determined to be in charge of her own life. After first developing cancer, Betty told me she decided it was time to take charge of her life. Prior to the cancer, she told me she was "trapped" in a "destructive" marriage. She also had one child who had serious mental incapacities; she had kept him at home for many years and cared for him. After she had surgery for cancer, she told me she came to realize that her future survival depended on her taking care of her own needs, not just those of others. At that time, Betty made the "very difficult" decision to place her son in an institution. Shortly thereafter, she and her husband of many years divorced at her request. She came to believe the marriage was one in which her needs were never considered, initially by both she and her husband. Later, as she came to value caring for herself, she said her husband refused to consider her needs and she demanded a divorce in order to effectively care for herself.

Betty said she believes she now can overcome her medical problems and can live with her pain, and she added that a lot of good things were happening in her life. She said she keeps busy and active, although she admitted to respecting her own limitations. She did not want to be dependent. In her opinion, pain patients need to "get up and get busy." She said she gets very disgusted with pain patients who will not do this. She states that the lidocaine infusions, in association with the meditation and relaxation training, have for the most part reduced her pain to what she defines as tolerable levels that she can live with.

Although she says she is happy with her physicians at the pain center, Betty was angry with former medical professionals and with her former employer and said she was going to control her own life from now on. She saw members of her family often and described her parents and siblings as very helpful and supportive. However, she told me she wanted "to escape my ethnic heritage" and become part of a "better educated" world. She is clearly making a deliberate effort to assimilate to the dominant Anglo-middle-class world she believes will offer her personal and professional advantages while retaining strong family ties.

Since her treatment for cancer and since obtaining her divorce, she completed a graduate program, obtaining a master's degree, and was actively seeking work in business administration when the study ended. Thus, while she had to give up her former employment as a nurse due to her pain, one of Betty's coping strategies was to retrain in a field in which she could function despite her pain and accompanying disability. Three years ago, Betty had received a financial settlement in her divorce case, which provided the financial resources needed to finance her graduate education and support her as she sought employment in her new field. At the end of the pain center study period, as the settlement resources were not unlimited, Betty was anxious to obtain employment in her new field.

Throughout the pain center study, Betty maintained an optimistic outlook and said she was able to deal effectively with her pain. She consistently said she saw herself as healthy and in control of her pain and her life.

Despite admitting to tiring easily, Betty always appeared energetic, well-dressed, and well-groomed and displayed a sense of humor. She maintained an active and "exciting" social life and was involved in a new relationship with a man who, she pointed out, was "a lot younger than me." Betty said she found this new relationship stimulating and fulfilling. She told me she believed a younger man was more likely to be willing to engage in a truly sharing relationship in which both partners' needs were met. The medical notes on her last exam before I left the center indicated that there was no evidence of recurrent cancer but cited the occurrence of more arthritic changes related to her former surgery and radiation therapy.

When I last saw Betty in early 1988, she was still optimistic and, despite a continued tiredness, she said she was doing well. The staff at the center seemed to share that view; the last notes from her file before I left the center at the end of February 1988 stated that "she continues to do well."

James, a forty-two-year-old divorced man, is our second Irish case study. He has a high school education but reported to us that he has some difficulty with reading and writing skills. When I met him in June of 1987, James described himself as a former artist but said he was no longer able to engage in his art due to arthritis in his hands. He is a New England native with family members in the area. He lives very near a sibling and several other relatives, yet did not feel he was close socially to most of them. He said he cuts himself off from others and does not like to have people visit him because he is very self-conscious about his pain and disability.

James's chronic pain began more than a decade ago when he survived a car accident, in which he suffered fractures of the skull, jaw, and neck, and other back injuries. He underwent an exploratory laminectomy after the accident, but no significant disk injury or disease was found. After the surgery he continued to have back and related leg pain, which left him dysfunctional. Since that time, although he has occasionally worked for brief periods, James has received his major form of financial support and funds for medical expenses through SSDI, Medicaid, and a state rehabilitation program.

After the initial accident, James underwent repeated diagnostic tests over the next several years, including a myelogram and other X-rays, but the record indicated no definitive findings. Throughout this period he was either partially or totally disabled from his pain, occasionally holding down jobs for brief periods until his pain and disability interfered with the work and he had to quit. In the early 1980s, James entered a live-in pain clinic in the New England area for six weeks. He was described in the hospital transcripts as a well-motivated patient who learned quickly and became significantly more functional by participating in the clinic's rehabilitation program.

Upon discharge he was defined as "physically able to do a full day's work if no excessive heavy lifting was involved." Despite his improvement, upon discharge, the clinic's staff noted that previous marital difficulties and a past reliance on alcohol as a way of dealing with difficulties could complicate his full recovery. The medical reports indicate that he tried to return to full-time employment after this discharge, but within a few weeks his back problems flared up again and upon examination he was found to have marked functional limitation in one leg associated with his back problems. New X-rays also showed some osteoarthritis of the spine. He was once again defined as totally disabled and given a narcotic medication for the pain. He was not considered a good candidate for repeat back surgery.

In 1984 he was referred through the state's rehabilitation program to the pain center for evaluation and treatment. In his early assessment at the center, the physicians noted severe osteoarthritis, posttraumatic neuropathy, tendonitis, low-back pain of unknown etiology, depression, and noncompliance with prescription drug directions. He also had some intestinal problems and reported increasing headaches.

Over the next several years James was treated with various modalities by the pain center and was referred by its physicians for repeated evaluations by specialists for his headaches, gastrointestinal problems, and arthritis. He alternately did somewhat better for a few weeks and then regressed. In late 1984 one physician noted that James's pain syndrome appeared almost intractable, given its duration and the heavy narcotics he had come to depend on for relief.

It also was noted that James had a deep mistrust of the medical profession inasmuch as he did not exhibit a healthy acceptance of new remedies. It was noted that he must decrease his dependence on methadone and improve his ability to engage in some sort of diversionary, pleasurable activity.

The medical record on James indicated attempts to taper off the methadone, followed within a few months by another increase in the methadone dose because of no relief from the pain severity. In 1985 James completed the center's stress-reduction program with a perfect attendance record. The instructor described him as "highly motivated" to work and noted that he was able to live with high levels of pain that "most people would give up on." Nonetheless, there was no permanent improvement in James's condition and over the next two years he continued to receive various treatments at the center and to be evaluated, reevaluated, and treated by a variety of medical and psychological specialists. The record shows repeated small improvements followed by regressions. Throughout the period James occasionally decreased the doses of methadone and other narcotic medications, later increasing them again.

By June 1987, when I first met him, he reported that his weight was at an all-time low and that he was only able to eat two days a week, the two days immediately after his weekly intravenous lidocaine treatment at the center. There was a continuing reliance on narcotic medications, and the methadone was increased again.

At this time, James was an extremely thin, tall man who displayed a great deal of pain behavior in the form of facial wincing, shaking and jerking of the body. During our first meeting he reported severe pain in his lower back, legs, neck, shoulders, and head, and defined himself as disabled. He was very depressed but extremely cooperative. He expressed extreme shame and distress regarding his disability and pain; he seldom went out in public and isolated himself in his apartment because of his fear that he might fall. On that first visit James told me several times that he just wanted to die because the pain and disability were more than he could bear.

He reported being in "excruciating pain almost all the time," the only exception being the first two to three days of each week immediately after his treatment with intravenous lidocaine, when his pain was partially relieved. James had a total pain intensity rating on the McGill Pain Questionnaire of 66, one of the highest scores in the study population.

I saw James weekly over the next nine months, often spending an hour or more talking to him during his intravenous lidocaine treatment. For the first five months he remained very discouraged, was unable to work, reported severe pain, continued to lose weight, and repeatedly told me he wished he were dead. He commented that if you cannot remain independent and care for yourself, "you are a useless human being and better off dead." He repeatedly expressed a sense of having no control and believed that his pain controlled his life. During the first interview with him, he said, "I don't have control over anything anymore. I let my hair grow long because it's the only place where I still have some control."

The center's psychologist stated, in a November 1987 psychological reevaluation on James, that the test results suggested "significant depression as an overlay to his current pain problem." It also was noted that during the reevaluation interview, James reported his current dosage of methadone was ineffective in reducing his pain and that he still was experiencing severe sleep disturbances. It also was noted he "lives a very isolated and sedentary lifestyle and has no recreational or social involvement. . . . [Furthermore, James] is severely dysfunctional, . . . has regressed considerably to an invalid role . . . [and] his life appears to be revolving around his pain problem."

Not long after this psychological reevaluation the center's staff decided to increase James's methadone. Shortly thereafter there was a dramatic improvement in his attitude and appearance. He also began using a TENS unit and said it helped his back and leg pain. He said by spring (1988) he intended to find a job or do some volunteer work. This was a very new perspective for him. He was strikingly better and very pleased with his new circumstances.

When the pain center study ended in February 1988, James still was doing fairly well. He continued to gain weight and was planning to return to part-time work in the near future. He was noticeably less depressed during the last three months of the study and did not return to his earlier practice of telling me he wished he were dead. He defined his quality of life as greatly improved and said he could function at this level and have a meaningful life as long as the pain center staff did not decrease the methadone. However, if the center's physicians did decrease James's methadone dosage again, it is doubtful that he would continue to do as well. Even if he was not physically addicted to his medication (which he probably was), it was clear from the interviews with him that he was psychologically dependent on it. In his view, the pain was so severe that only large doses of methadone could decrease it enough to make life bearable.

After more than ten years of chronic pain and narcotic use, James appears to be involved in a permanent cycle of drug dependency and social isolation, with brief periods of some improvement, which never seem to last for more than a few months. It is clear that James believes his pain can only be controlled and his life made bearable through drug use. Thus, James is totally dependent on this external factor and on the physicians and other health-care providers who make possible his access to these prescription medications. Without these external forces, James cannot sustain a lifestyle that is meaningful and worthwhile to him.

James and Betty demonstrate the diversity found within specific ethnic groups. Their cases demonstrate the need for studies that look at intra-ethnic-group—as well as inter-ethnic-group—differences in the chronic pain experience and show that stereotyping of patients on the basis of ethnic background is always inappropriate.

QUANTITATIVE FINDINGS OF PAIN RESPONSE VARIATION

The case studies described in the preceding pages demonstrate considerable diversity in patients' responses to chronic pain and in their abilities to adapt to the pain experience and once again have meaningful and happy lives. What specific factors are associated with the differences in patients' abilities to cope with the chronic pain experience? To determine what those factors are, in the quantitative section of this chapter three major research questions will be addressed: (1) Are there *statistically significant* differences in pain responses in the pain center population and, if so, what variables are associated with the variation? (2) Are there statistically significant differences in responses to chronic pain in the pain center population which are related to ethnic identity when other variables which affect response are controlled? (3) Are there statistically significant variations in pain responses *within ethnic groups*? If so, what cultural, sociodemographic, psychological, or biological factors are associated with those differences?

Inter-Ethnic-Group Variation in Pain Responses

In the one-way analysis of variances (ANOVAs), there were significant inter-ethnic-group variations in the pain center study population in behavioral, attitudinal, psychological and emotional responses to chronic pain. After completing the ANOVAs, multiple regression analyses were performed on each response area. In each regression equation, the independent variables that showed significant relationships to the specific response area in the ANOVAs were included. Table 5.1 presents only inter-ethnic-group differences in pain responses that remained significant in the regressions. (For those readers interested in reviewing the multiple regression tables, they are located in appendix F, table F.3.)

Behavioral response: Significant differences appeared among several ethnic groups regarding the necessity to stop normal work inside and outside the home (work stoppage) (table 5.1). A Duncan's Multiple Range test determined that the significant differences were between the Anglo American group and both the Italian and French Canadian groups, and between the Latino group and the Polish, Irish, and French Canadian groups. (Education, workers' compensation status, and gender all also remained significantly related to differences in work stoppage in regressions [see appendix F]. Men reported higher work stoppage levels than women, those receiving workers' compensation reported higher work stoppage than those who were not, and those with higher education levels reported less work stoppage.)

As to self-reported expression of pain, expressiveness was highest in the Latino group (a mean of 15.3 out of a possible aggregated score of 20). The Italian group had the second-highest expressiveness mean (12.7), while the Anglo Americans had the lowest at 10.3 (table 5.1).

There were no ethnic-group differences, however, in the behavioral category, "total interference in all daily activities," which was determined by adding each patient's scores on all of the items on the activity-interference chart of the pain control center's admission questionnaire (appendix E), including sleep, eating, sports, job, social activities, household chores, driving, walking, and sex ($F = .60$, Sig. $= .63$). There was, though, a significant difference in interference in all daily activities between the three age groups in the total study population: the oldest age group (age 61 and up) had the lowest interference mean of 10.5, the youngest group (ages 15–40) had the highest interference mean of 21.2, while the middle-aged group

Table 5.1. Statistically Significant Inter-Ethnic-Group Variations in Behavioral, Psychological, and Attitudinal Responses

	Ethnic Groups						
Response Area	Anglo American	Latino	Italian	French Canadian	Irish	Polish	F-ratio
Stopped Work[a]							3.60**
Mean	5.1	7.3	6.5	6.0	6.0	5.1	
SD	2.7	1.4	2.3	2.2	2.5	2.4	
Expressiveness[b]							7.44**
Mean	10.3	15.3	12.7	12.0	11.3	10.9	
SD	3.3	3.3	4.0	3.5	3.8	3.3	
Sought Friends' and Family's Advice							3.73*
Mean	1.4	2.7	1.8	1.6	1.6	1.6	
SD	1.3	1.4	1.2	1.3	1.2	1.6	
Pain = Unhappiness[c]							9.97**
Mean	1.8	3.3	2.6	2.1	1.6	1.1	
SD	1.2	1.2	1.5	1.1	1.1	0.1	
Worry[b]							7.60*
Mean	5.4	8.7	6.6	5.7	5.4	5.3	
SD	2.7	1.8	2.3	2.9	2.8	2.8	
Tension[b]							3.01**
Mean	3.0	3.8	3.4	3.0	3.3	2.8	
SD	1.3	0.6	1.0	1.2	0.9	1.0	
Anger[b]							3.61**
Mean	2.6	3.7	2.9	2.7	2.6	2.4	
SD	1.4	0.8	1.3	1.2	1.3	1.1	

(Continued on next page)

Table 5.1. (*Cont'd.*)

Response Area	Ethnic Groups						F-ratio
	Anglo American	Latino	Italian	French Canadian	Irish	Polish	
Health Attitude[d]							Chi-square 21.87**
Healthy	60%	17%	47%	59%	45%	45%	
Unhealthy/Disabled	40%	83%	53%	41%	55%	55%	

SD = Standard Deviation

*$p < .05$

**$p < .01$

[a]Degree to which patient had to stop work (inside and outside home) due to pain; higher score indicates greatest work stoppage.

[b]Pain-related worry, tension, etc.; higher score indicates greater degree.

[c]Does patient believe that as long as pain persists his or her life will be unhappy? Higher scores indicate agreement that life will remain unhappy.

[d]Patient asked to define self as healthy or unhealthy/disabled.

Note: Since many response scores are an aggregated score from several questions, the highest possible score varies by item.

had the highest interference mean of 21.2, while the middle-aged group (ages 41–60) had a mean of 19.7 ($F = 32.31, p < .01$).

Attitudinal response: Several attitudinal response areas showed significant differences among the ethnic groups. For example, patients were asked if, and how strongly, they agreed with the statement: "As long as I am in pain, I will never have a fulfilling and happy life." The Latinos had the highest mean, indicating stronger agreement; the Italians, the second-highest; and the Polish the lowest (table 5.1).

In another attitudinal area, patients were asked their attitudes toward their current health status,[1] using the categories of "healthy" or "unhealthy/disabled." A chi-square cross-tabulation showed significant differences in the distributions of the two health-status attitudes across the six ethnic groups (table 5.1), although there was no significant difference in the distributions of the three main *diagnostic* categories among them (table 3.1). Sixty percent of the Anglo Americans and 59% of French Canadians defined themselves as healthy, while only 17% of Latinos, 45% of Polish, 45% of Irish, and 47% of Italians defined themselves as healthy.

Two other attitudinal response areas showed *no* significant ethnic differences—patients' reported beliefs concerning support from family and friends during their pain experiences ($F = 1.07$, Sig. $= .38$) and patients' attitudes regarding their ability to eventually overcome their pain ($F = .95$, Sig. $= .45$).

Psychological/emotional response: Several psychological/emotional response areas, including differences in degree of anger, tension, and worry associated with pain (table 5.1), showed significant intergroup differences. The Latino group had the highest mean in each of these response areas, the Italian group the second-highest, and the Polish group the lowest.

In regard to *care and treatment actions*, significant differences appeared in the degree to which patients asked for and used the advice of family and friends regarding pain treatments. The Latino group reported seeking and using advice most often, the Anglo American group least

---

1. Patients' attitudes toward their health status have been found to be important as predictors of adjustment to chronic pain. Jensen and Karoly (1991) found that those chronic pain "patients who believed themselves to be disabled by the pain demonstrated significantly lower levels of activity and psychological well-being and higher levels of professional services utilization" (128). Thus, this was an especially important attitude to assess in chronic pain populations; however, Jensen and Karoly made no mention of the possible influence of cultural or ethnic background on patients' attitudes toward their health status.

often (table 5.1). A Duncan's Multiple Range test revealed that Latinos sought advice more often than any of the other groups except the Polish. This finding was understandable, as the Latin American cultural tradition, much more than mainstream Anglo American tradition, emphasizes personal relations and the establishment of such networks to provide support and advice.

No significant interethnic differences were revealed in patients' reported compliance with physicians' directions on medications or treatments ($F = 2.11$, Sig. = .07). There also were no ethnic differences in whether or not the patient immediately sought the care of a medical doctor when the pain began.

There was a difference in seeking the care of a doctor immediately related to workers' compensation status. Those receiving compensation were significantly more likely to seek care immediately than those who weren't. In the ANOVA, the group receiving compensation had a mean for seeking immediate care of 3.7 (out of a possible 4.0), while the non–workers' compensation group had a mean of 3.2 ($F = 8.39$, $p < .01$). The workers' compensation difference remained in regression analysis when the other independent variables (LOC style and pain duration) related to variation in seeking care in the ANOVAs were controlled (appendix F, table F.4). However, when workers' compensation was controlled for, neither LOC style or pain duration remained significant. The likely explanation for this relationship between workers' compensation status and seeking immediate care from a doctor is the gate-keeping function assigned to physicians in the U.S. workers' compensation system. Workers cannot receive workers' compensation benefits unless their injuries are assessed, diagnosed, and documented by a physician.

Intra-Ethnic-Group Variation in Pain Responses

Significant variations in pain response also appeared *within* several of the pain center ethnic groups. (It should be noted that the sample size of the Polish group, $N = 28$, made statistically valid intragroup comparisons difficult; for those categories where valid comparisons could be made, with the exception of two differences related to workers' compensation status, few variations were found, due perhaps to actual group homogeneity or, obviously, to small sample size.) Most frequently, intragroup response variations were related to degree of heritage consistency, patient's generation, LOC style, age, socioeconomic status (SES), and workers' compensation status.

Heritage consistency was related to response variation within each of the Latino, Italian, French Canadian, and Irish groups. For each group a Pearson's Correlation Coefficient was used to determine whether there was a correlation between heritage consistency and variation in total interference in daily activities.

In the Italian and Irish groups, high heritage consistency correlated with significantly lower levels of total interference with daily activities (table 5.2). In the French Canadian and Irish groups, high heritage consistency related significantly to lower degrees of depression and correlated with higher degrees of reported social support from family and friends during the pain experience. Such high degrees of social support may well have helped to lessen the depression associated with the pain.

There was also a correlation between heritage consistency and support of family and friends within the Latino group. Again, high heritage consistency correlated with reports of high degrees of family/friend support during the pain experience. Latinos with high heritage consistency also reported a significantly higher degree of expressiveness of their pain (table 5.2).

Generation also related to intragroup variations. Using a Pearson Correlation, it was determined that in the Latino group, the later the generation, the higher the fear level (thus, being first- or second-generation U.S.-mainland-born correlated with higher fear levels associated with the pain experience than found in the immigrant generation) (table 5.2). Given that U.S.-mainland-born Latinos reported less strong ties to the local Latino community than did the immigrants and that, as mentioned above, heritage consistency correlated with a support network of family/friends, it appears that strong social support may have helped reduce the fears of the immigrant group.

These findings reflect the Latino orientation to life, which views the family as the paramount mediating institution between the individual and his/her social and physical reality (Sanchez-Ayendez 1984). Within this orientation, interdependence underlies family relations, a value that ensues from the belief that individuals are not capable of doing everything and, therefore, should rely on others for assistance (Bastida 1979:70–71).

According to this study, generation in the Latino group also correlated with degree of expressiveness: the later the generation, the less the degree of expressiveness (table 5.2), possibly owing to assimilation into the Anglo American ethic of stoicism.

In the French Canadian group, generation was related to differences in degree of tension associated with the pain; the later the generation, the

Table 5.2. Statistically Significant Intra-Ethnic-Group Variations in Pain Response

| | Ethnic Group | | | |
	Latino	Italian	French Canadian	Irish
Response Areas				
Generation and Expressiveness				
PCC	.45			
p	.01			
Fear				
PCC	.38			
p	.02			
Tension				
PCC			.29	
p			.03	
Support[a]				
PCC			−.25	
p			.05	
Heritage Consistency and Expressiveness				
PCC	.38			
p	.03			
Support[a]				
PCC	.33	.44	.32	.49
p	.00	.01	.02	.00
Total Interference[b]				
PCC		−.44		−.38
p		.01		.01
Depression				
PCC			.31	−.31
p			.03	.02

PCC = Pearson Correlation Coefficients
[a]Degree of family and friends' support reported by patient.
[b]Total interference in all daily activities.

greater the degree of tension (table 5.2). Again, the likely explanation is that successive generations decrease their ties to the local ethnic community, and this may result in less social support, which could increase the patient's tension level. In fact, French Canadians also showed correlations between both generation and degree of heritage consistency and degree of family/friend support. As the generation ascended, reported social support descended, while as heritage consistency increased, so did social support (table 5.2).

    LOC style related to significant variations in emotional response to pain (tension, anger, and/or fear) within the Anglo American, Italian,

French Canadian, and Latino groups (table 5.3). In the Italian, French Canadian, and Anglo American groups, means for anger, fear, tension, or depression were significantly higher in the external LOC subgroups. In a similar manner, in the Latino group, the internal style subgroup reported less depression and less work stoppage than the external group. In addition, 40% of members of the Latino internal subgroup defined themselves as healthy, while 100% of members of the external subgroup defined themselves as unhealthy and/or disabled. Consistent with the idea that members of the external LOC subgroup perceived that control over their life circumstances rested outside of themselves, among Latinos the members of the external LOC subgroup were significantly more likely to seek the advice of family and friends concerning care and treatment than were

Table 5.3. Intra-Ethnic-Group Variations in Pain Responses by Locus-of-Control (LOC) Style

Response Area	Internal LOC Style		External LOC Style		
	Mean	Standard Deviation	Mean	Standard Deviation	T
Degree of Anger					
Italian	2.3	1.4	3.7	0.5	−3.3*
French Canadian	2.3	1.2	3.4	0.9	−2.6*
Degree of Fear					
Italian	1.1	0.5	2.5	1.5	−3.1**
French Canadian	1.6	1.2	2.8	1.3	−2.6*
Degree of Depression					
Italian	2.7	1.4	3.8	0.4	−2.8*
Latino	3.4	1.1	4.0	0.2	4.06*
Degree of Tension					
Anglo American	2.3	1.2	3.8	0.3	−2.5*
Seeks Treatment Advice[a]					
Latino	1.7	1.4	3.0	1.4	4.71*
Work Stoppage[b]					
Latino	6.3	1.6	7.6	7.6	5.88*
	Healthy	Unhealthy/ Disabled	Healthy	Unhealthy/ Disabled	Chi-square[d]
View of Health Status[c] (% in each category)					
Latino	40%	60%	0%	100%	5.58*

*$p < .05$
**$p < .01$
[a]Degree to which patient seeks advice from family and friends concerning treatment actions.
[b]Degree to which patient had to stop work inside and outside the home due to the pain.
[c]Patient asked to define health status as healthy or unhealthy/disabled.
[d]Using Fisher's Exact.

members of the internal LOC subgroup. Clearly, with individuals in these four groups, a sense that one has control, or at least some control, over one's life circumstances has had a positive affect on the patient's responses to his or her pain experience.

Among Anglo Americans, Italians, and Irish, *age* related to significant intragroup differences regarding interference in daily activities as a whole. In each ethnic group the youngest age group (20–40 years) had the highest or next-to-highest total interference mean (out of a possible 44), while the oldest group (61 years and older) consistently had the lowest mean in all three ethnic groups (table 5.4). At least in part, age-group differences regarding total interference in daily activities were likely the result of most members of the oldest age group being retired and thus not having employment obligations. Other significant relationships between age and intra-ethnic-group pain-response variations are presented in table 5.4. In each instance, the oldest age group seemed to better adjust to the pain, were more likely to seek advice of members of their social networks, and reported less behavioral interference and less anger and tension related to the pain experience than the two younger groups.

The qualitative data suggest that one of the factors involved in these age differences is that those who are retired (and thus older) are less stressed about their pain because they do not have the day-to-day worry that when the pain is bad they will be unable to meet employment or childcare obligations. If retired people have a bad pain day, they simply "take it easy." They can do this without fear of job loss or of not finishing employment tasks. For those who are younger and still employed (or have child-care responsibilities), a bad pain day leads to many problems because important obligations cannot be met—thus, the person experiences additional tension and stress.

SES related to several significant intragroup differences in responses among all groups except the Polish group, whose size was too small to allow valid intragroup analysis—except in the case of education, which showed no significant correlations. Only the differences related to education and income levels will be presented here. They are reflective of similar response differences found in data analyses related to occupation categories.

Among Anglo Americans, French Canadians, Irish, and Latinos, education or income level related to significant differences in current employment status or degree of reported stoppage of normal work inside or outside the home. As educational or income level rose, the percentage of each group still employed rose also; or as education level went up, degree of work stoppage went down (table 5.5). Obviously, these differences related in part to conditions of employment. Professional college-

Table 5.4. Intra-Ethnic-Group Variations in Pain Responses by Age

	20–40 years		41–60 years		61+ years		
	Mean	SD	Mean	SD	Mean	SD	F-ratio
Anglo American							
Total							
Interference[a]	22.2	7.3	20.9	6.7	7.3	10.8	20.34**
Work							
Stoppage[a]	4.7	2.6	6.4	2.4	1.5	1.0	6.43**
Degree of Anger[a]	2.9	1.1	3.0	1.3	.8	.5	6.55**
Italian							
Total							
Interference[a]	19.9	12.2	22.2	6.1	8.5	9.8	7.30**
Seeks Advice of Family & Friends	1.8	1.3	1.1	1.1	2.5	1.1	3.22**
Thinks About What Was Done to Deserve Pain	1.9	1.6	1.0	.8	3.6	1.1	10.73**
Irish							
Total							
Interference[a]	19.9	8.7	21.1	8.7	7.3	9.9	10.24**
French Canadian							
Belief One Can Overcome Pain	3.3	.9	3.1	1.6	2.1	1.8	3.51*
Degree of Tension	3.6	.8	3.3	.9	1.6	1.4	11.46*

Note: Many response scores are an aggregated score from several questions, so the highest possible score varies by item.

SD = Standard Deviation.

*$p < .05$

**$p < .01$

[a]Higher score indicates greater degree of overall interference in all daily activities, or work stoppage, anger, or fear.

Table 5.5. Intra-Ethnic-Group Variations in Pain Responses by Socioeconomic Status

Response Area	Income Category				F-ratio
	$0–$7,000	$7,001–$18,000	$18,001–$28,000	$28,001 +	
Fear[a]					
Anglo-American					4.41**
Mean	3.0	1.6	1.4	0.9	
SD	1.5	0.9	1.1	0.4	
French Canadian					4.32**
Mean	3.5	1.7	2.8	1.7	
SD	1.2	1.0	1.2	1.5	
Work Stoppage[a]					
Irish					4.41**
Mean	7.4	6.5	3.6	5.0	
SD	1.4	2.1	3.2	1.7	
Latino					3.02*
Mean	7.6	7.4	7.5	4.0	
SD	1.0	1.2	0.7	0.0	
Unhappiness[a]					
Irish					3.12*
Mean	2.3	1.2	1.5	1.0	
SD	1.3	1.0	0.9	0.0	
Anger[a]					
Italian					5.43**
Mean	3.2	3.5	1.5		
SD	1.3	1.5	0.8		
Tension[a]					
Latino					4.03*
Mean	3.7	4.0	2.5	2.0	
SD	0.4	0.0	2.1	0.0	

(Continued on next page)

Table 5.5. (Cont'd.)

	Education Level				
	Less than 12 years	High school graduate	Some college	College degree	Chi-square
Presently Employed					
Anglo American					19.2*
Yes	8%	27%	38%	44%	
No	92%	73%	64%	56%	
French Canadian					19.0*
Yes	9%	23%	26%	66%	
No	91%	77%	74%	34%	

SD = Standard Deviation
*p < .05
**p < .01
[a]Higher score indicates greater degree of fear, work stoppage, unhappiness, anger, or tension.

educated and well-paid subjects who did not have to engage in manual labor and who often had worktime flexibility were more likely to still be employed. In contrast, less-educated working-class unskilled and semi-skilled subjects' employment conditions more likely involved rigid forty-hour-a-week schedules and required manual labor, both of which were insurmountable barriers for those with chronic pain and thus caused work stoppage.

There were also significant intragroup variations in both the Anglo American and French Canadian groups in the degree of fear associated with the pain by income level. Not surprisingly, in both ethnic groups the lowest income group had the highest level of fear associated with the pain. Similar emotional response variations were found in the Irish, Latino, and Italian groups, where higher-income-category groups reported less unhappiness, fear, or tension (table 5.5).

Thus, within the ethnic groups, the less-educated, lower-income groups consistently reported higher degrees of emotional responses than did the higher-paid and better-educated groups. As many patients in lower-income and less-educated groups expressed fears and anxiety related to the financial troubles associated with their pain problems—including fears of losing workers' compensation benefits and fears of not being able to support their families—it is likely that those with adequate income had less to fear from an economic perspective.

Workers' compensation status also related to significant intra-ethnic-group differences in response in several groups (although there were no significant relationships between worker's compensation status and pain intensity). In the Latino and Polish groups, those receiving workers' compensation reported a significantly higher level of total interference in daily activities (table 5.6). In the Italian and French Canadian groups, compensation status related to significant differences in interference with normal work inside and outside the home. In each case, the group receiving workers' compensation had a significantly higher work-stoppage mean than the noncompensation group.

In addition, among Latinos and Italians, compensation status related to significant differences in immediately seeking the care of a doctor, with the group receiving compensation being significantly more likely to seek immediate care than the non-compensation group. In another care and treatment area, in the Anglo American and Latino groups those receiving workers' compensation were more likely to report taking medication exactly as directed by their physician than noncompensation patients (table 5.6).

There was a significant variation among Anglo Americans in the belief that they would be able to overcome the pain related to workers'

Table 5.6. Intra-Ethnic-Group Variations in Pain Responses by
Workers' Compensation Status

Response Area	Receiving compensation		Not receiving compensation		
	Mean	Standard Deviation	Mean	Standard Deviation	F-ratio
Follows doctor's orders in taking medications[a]					
Anglo American	3.5	0.5	2.6	1.3	4.8*
Latino	3.5	0.9	2.5	1.4	4.4*
Belief that one can overcome pain[b]					
Anglo American	2.1	1.1	3.3	0.9	9.0**
Total interference in daily activities[c]					
Latino	23.9	7.4	15.0	11.5	9.0**
Polish	22.3	6.0	15.8	9.2	4.6*
Sought immediate care of doctor					
Latino	4.0	1.4	2.7	1.2	9.9**
Italian	4.0	0.0	3.0	1.2	7.3**
Degree of work stoppage[c]					
Italian	7.5	1.3	5.5	2.8	4.7*
French Canadian	7.4	1.2	5.1	2.1	17.2*
Degree of Unhappiness					
Polish	1.5	0.5	0.6	0.1	7.4*

*p < .05
**p < .01
[a]Higher score indicates patient reports following doctor's directions when taking medications.
[b]Higher score indicates stronger belief in ability to overcome the pain.
[c]Higher score indicates greater degree of overall interference in all daily activities or work stoppage.

compensation status. Those receiving compensation were less likely to believe they could eventually overcome the pain than the group receiving no compensation. In the Polish group, workers' compensation also related to significant differences in unhappiness, with the compensation group being more likely to agree that chronic pain meant a life of unhappiness than the noncompensation group (table 5.6).

The significant relationships between workers' compensation status and patients' behavioral and attitudinal responses were understandable because the qualitative data showed that many patients at the pain center were initially denied compensation by their insurer for job-related injuries. In case after case, patients told of initial denial followed by two to three years of fighting with the state workers' compensation boards, and in some cases going to the courts, for their benefits. Generally those who finally appealed the decision through the courts ultimately won their cases. However, during the two to three years of appeals they received no income and suffered severe financial hardship. In several cases, patients lost their homes or apartments and had to move their spouse and children into the homes of extended family members, and these patients experienced severe psychosocial stress during that period.

For those who ultimately won their cases, the stress did not end with the workers' compensation board's or court's decision. The adversarial relationship established by the process instilled a fear of engaging in any physical activity. Several such patients told me they did not dare to go outside their homes to walk or do light chores for fear of workers' compensation insurance agents being in the area to "spy" on them. These patients came to fear that any physical activity on their part would be used against them by the workers' compensation insurance carrier in an effort to take away their hard-won benefits.

SUMMARY AND DISCUSSION

Quantitative analyses showed that the most frequent and consistent differences in pain intensity and responses in the New England pain control center study population were related to variation in ethnic identity and LOC style. In the total pain center population or within one or more ethnic groups, an internal LOC style was associated with significantly lower levels of work stoppage, unhappiness, anger, worry, fear, depression, or tension, and those with an internal style were significantly more likely to define their health status as healthy.

Furthermore, the study found a significant relationship between LOC style and ethnic identity, as there was a significant difference in the distributions of the two styles across the ethnic groups. With the exception of the Anglo American group, ethnic or cultural identity was a predictor of LOC style. As it is impossible for LOC style to influence ethnic identity, probably ethnic background (i.e., socialization, social learning, and psychosocial experiences as a member of the group) affects the LOC style one develops. (There were no significant relationships between the distribution of the two LOC styles and the other sociodemographic variables in the pain center study, including age, gender, SES, and religion.)

Even when LOC style was controlled for, ethnic background still was associated with significant pain response variations at the pain center. The ethnic pattern was consistent: the Latino group had the highest intensity mean, the greatest interference with work and social activities, the highest degree of emotional and psychological stress, and the highest pain expressiveness; the Italian group was second-highest in each of these categories; and either the Polish or Anglo American group was always lowest in each category.

The Irish and French Canadian groups did not differ significantly from each other in pain intensity means, rarely differed significantly from each other in pain responses, and often did not differ significantly from the Anglo American group. However, the Irish and French Canadians did generally differ significantly from the Latinos and often from the Italians and Polish. Thus the analyses show that the most pronounced interethnic differences in pain intensity and response (i.e., the highest and lowest means) usually were associated with the Latino, Italian, and Polish groups. These three ethnic groups had the highest means for heritage consistency, indicating close ethnic ties and lifestyles reflective of their ethnic heritages. These three groups also are the only groups that had majorities in the immigrant or first- or second-generation U.S.-born categories. Therefore, in the New England study population, the ethnic groups that appeared least assimilated to Anglo American culture showed the greatest variation in pain intensity and response.

Furthermore, the intragroup analyses demonstrated that *within* several ethnic groups, those who were immigrants or first-generation U.S.-born, who had high degrees of heritage consistency, and who believed they had the strong social support of family and friends reported less severe (although not necessarily less expressive) responses to the pain in several areas. In this study population then, generation and degree of heritage consistency both appeared to modify the effect of ethnic affiliation on the pain experience, probably because both were related to degree of social support, and social support has often been shown to relate to variation in health status (House, Landis, and Umberson 1990; Jacobson 1987).

The quantitative intragroup analyses also show that while the chronic pain experience may be affected by one's cultural background, clearly the individual's life experiences, cognitive perceptions, coping style, social roles and relationships, and socioeconomic circumstances can contribute to differences between individuals within a specific cultural or ethnic group. (The intragroup variations clearly demonstrate the inappropriateness and dangers of ethnic or cultural stereotyping, and illustrate the need to evaluate each patient as an individual.)

The quantitative segment of the pain center study also reveals very little association between diagnoses or types of medications currently being taken for pain and patients' reported pain intensity levels or their abilities to adapt to the chronic pain. Other studies of chronic pain populations have also found that there are often no significant relationships between diagnosis and/or types of medications being taken for pain and variations in reported chronic pain intensity and responses (McNeil, Sinkora, and Levavitt 1986; Jensen and Karoly 1991; Stenger 1992; Turk 1993). In this multiethnic comparison, the factors associated with an ability to successfully adapt to pain and once again have a life defined by the pain sufferer as worthwhile were most often cultural, psychological/ cognitive, social, and economic factors.

The case studies show—at the microlevel—how cultural meanings, beliefs, attitudes, and standards for behavior, as well as socioeconomic circumstances and psychological characteristics, affect pain sufferers' ability to adapt to the chronic pain. The case studies also demonstrate that the cultural, political, and economic context of the health-care setting has an impact on the complex human chronic pain experience.

Finally, while it appears that differences in attitudes, values, beliefs, and standards among several of the ethnic groups in the New England study related to pain intensity and response variation, the issue of the emigration experience of the Latinos must be addressed. The majority of Latino patients at the pain center had been on the U.S. mainland for two to five years (having migrated from Puerto Rico); they are mostly not fluent in English and have an average education level of 8.7 years. When chronic pain is added to these social constraints, it is not hard to imagine that these Latinos will experience high degrees of stress, tension, and worries.

The small size of the nonimmigrant Latino group (9 out of 44) made it difficult to clearly establish whether there were significant intragroup differences in the Latino group related to generation or migration status. In the quantitative analyses, the major *response differences* that appeared to be related to generation were in degree of expressiveness of the pain and degree of interference with work. There were no *statistically significant differences in pain intensity* within the Latino group related to generation, language spoken in the childhood home, or degree of heritage consistency (although the group with high heritage consistency did have a lower intensity mean, the difference did not reach statistical significance). Given the small size of the nonimmigrant group, however, these intragroup findings must be viewed with caution. Therefore, it is possible that some of the significant differences in pain intensity and response between the Latinos and the other five groups may be the result of the recent emigration component of the ethnic experience of Latinos. For members of the other four non–Anglo American groups, recent emigration is not part of their current ethnic experience since the majority have been in the United States for one to three generations and speak English fluently.

I believed it was important to determine the role of cultural influences on chronic pain in Latinos without the influence of their recent emigration experience, because many of the differences in the pain center population were between the Latinos and the other five groups. Therefore, since 1990, as the First Principal Investigator on an NSF- and NIH-funded study in Puerto Rico, an attempt has been made to more clearly analyze the effects of cultural orientation and the migration experience on chronic pain. Chapter 6 will present data on the native Puerto Ricans and their chronic pain experiences. Chapter 7 will present a comparison of the native Puerto Ricans and the Latinos in the New England study in order to determine the effects of both culture and migration on the pain experience, and a cross-cultural comparison of the native Puerto Ricans and the Anglo Americans also will be presented in order to further assess *cultural* influences on the chronic pain experience.

CHAPTER 6

THE PUERTO RICAN STUDY

INTRODUCTION

The first inhabitants of Puerto Rico were the Taino Indians. In the early 1500s the island was colonized by the Spanish, and many Taino Indians were enslaved. Subsequently, many natives died from European disease epidemics or during forced labor. Thus, colonization had a devastating effect on the native Taino population (Canino and Canino 1993:467). According to Canino and Canino, after a long period of Spanish colonial rule, by the mid-1800s "the people on the island developed a growing separatist fervor" (468). In addition, Spain was experiencing financial burdens related to its colonies and, in 1897, the "Spanish Prime Minister declared Puerto Rico an autonomous state, allowing the Spanish-appointed governor only restricted powers" (468).

However, this was short-lived, as in 1889, during the Spanish-American War, United States soldiers landed on the island and Puerto Rico became a protectorate of the United States (Canino and Canino 1993:468). Since that time, the island's political groups have often been divided into pro-American and anti-American factions (469). Due to the island's particular history, Puerto Rican cultural heritage has four major influences: Indian, Spanish, African, and American (Ahearn 1979:4).

Today, Puerto Rico is a commonwealth of the United States with some degree of self government, and can elect its own island officials, including the highest ranking official, the governor. Puerto Ricans are United States citizens with rights to unrestricted migration to the mainland. Despite citizenship status, Puerto Ricans on the island have no voting representatives in Congress, although they do have one nonvoting representative (Weisman 1990:30). Puerto Ricans on the island do not pay U.S. federal income taxes, and the island does not receive the same level of social welfare as the U.S. states. However, "commonwealth status carries benefits, too. . . . [U.S.] companies establishing business on the island are given federal tax incentives that they could not receive in a state" (Marshall 1991:82).

The political status of Puerto Rico, in relationship to the United States, is still hotly debated on the island and among Puerto Ricans who have migrated to the mainland United States. In fact today, the island's main "three political parties are themselves largely defined by their respective positions on the [future political] status question" (Marshall 1991:83). Twice in recent years, there has been an island plebiscite to assess the public's preference for formal U.S. statehood status, continuation of commonwealth status, or independence. The results of the most recent (November 1993) referendum showed that a narrow majority preferred the present commonwealth status to statehood; however, this vote was very close and another vote may occur in the not-too-distant future.

The population of Puerto Rico was approximately 3.3 million in 1987 (Departamento de Salud 1989; Canino and Canino 1993). At that time, over 2.5 million other Puerto Ricans resided on the U.S. mainland (Canino and Canino 1993:471). As Reyes and Inclan (1991) note, "most Puerto Rican who migrate to the United States [mainland] do so for economic reasons" (1). Since the late 1940s, there has been rapid development of the island's tourist industry and industrialization of the island associated with "Operation Bootstrap," which included tax incentives to attract U.S. industries to the island (Rodriguez 1991:11-12). Nonetheless, the current rate of unemployment on the island is quite high, 14.4% in 1989 (Departamento de Trabajo 1989), and a substantial segment of the island population receives some form of public assistance: according to the Departamento Servicios Sociales, 67% received public assistance income in 1988 (as quoted in Canino and Canino 1993:471).

Canino and Canino (1993) note that "several factors that characterize Puerto Rican history . . . have created particular difficulties for Puerto Ricans. The continuous impact of a variety of cultures and races, consistent economic difficulties and transitions, and the powerful influence of colonizing countries have created sociocultural, economic, and political stresses" (472). These stressors include displacement of agricultural workers from their land, rapid increases in urban populations, and urban poverty, which have led to substantial mental-health, social, and economic stresses; environmental damage; various forms of socioeconomic and racial discrimination; and continued political dissension concerning the island's future. In addition, back-and-forth migration between the island and U.S. mainland often has put additional stress on

Puerto Rican families, including some lessening of daily support to elderly extended family members (Canino and Canino 1993:473; Sanchez-Ayendez 1993).

Sanchez-Ayendez (1993) notes that "not all aspects of culture change at the same time. Some, as those related to worldviews, family relations, and male/female roles in the domestic and public spheres of life, are more resistant to change. . . . In the real world, social and cultural change do not necessarily go hand-in-hand" (2-3).

Although there has been a degree of Americanization on the island, despite over ninety years of American rule Puerto Rico remains distinctive culturally (Zayas and Palleja 1988:260), and a clear preference for the Spanish language and Spanish as the language of instruction in the public schools remain important symbols of Puerto Rican identity (Rodriguez 1991:17). Studies indicate that Puerto Ricans prefer to identify themselves as Puerto Rican rather than American (Sanchez-Ayendez 1988; Zayas and Palleja 1988:260; Rodriguez 1991). The results of the 1993 referendum also show a majority of Puerto Ricans still prefer the present commonwealth status to statehood.

While acknowledging the existence of substantial diversity among Puerto Ricans, especially differences related to island or mainland residence, place of birth, and socioeconomic status (Morales Carrion 1983; Robles et al. 1982; Szalay and Diaz-Guerrero 1985; Duany 1988-89; Rogler, Cortez, and Malgady 1991; Schensul, Nieves, and Martinez 1982; Canino and Canino 1980; Rodriguez 1991; Harwood 1977), the literature has identified certain cultural values common to many Puerto Ricans. These widely shared values include "personalismo," "the need to relate to people and not to institutions" (Canino and Canino 1993:480). A related value which has been identified in the literature is that of allocentrism—or collectivism—where the needs, values, and goals of the group are emphasized over that of the individual. Marin and Triandis (1985) maintain that "an important element of the difference between Anglos and Hispanics/Latin Americans seems to be the emphasis Latino Americans and Hispanics place on their reference group as contrasted with the individualism present among non-Hispanics" (98).

Another value common to many Puerto Ricans is "respeto," which "implies generalized deference in all social interactions " (Lauria 1964, as quoted in Sanchez-Ayendez 1988:243); "it also involves a variety of deferential acts or rituals that are relevant to specific types of social relations" (243).

The continued importance of a cultural value on "familismo" is also mentioned in the literature. Familismo (or familialism) involves strong identification with and attachment to nuclear and extended families; a high value on giving and receiving family support; stress on family interdependence, loyalty, reciprocity, and solidarity; and the continuation of strong parental control over offspring (Bastida 1979; Canino and Canino 1993; Canino et al. 1987; Marin and VanOss Marin 1991; Sanchez-Ayendez 1988). Some lessening of this parental control has been noted in mainland families who assimilate to more symmetrical family relations of Anglo American culture (Canino and Canino 1993; Canino et al. 1987). In addition, daily support of elderly family members may vary among island Puerto Ricans in relationship to migration of adult children to the mainland. However, my research and that of others suggest that other extended family members, such as brothers, sisters, nieces, and nephews, may provide support in the absence of daughters, sons, or other family members (Sanchez-Ayendez 1993). Sanchez-Ayendez (1992, 1993) notes that while caregiving is dynamic and changes through time and the ways in which familial support is offered have not remained unaltered, extended families still provide much of the care and support of the Puerto Rican elderly.

The retention of a value on traditional Puerto Rican gender roles, with some variation from such roles related to socioeconomic class and long-term stays on the mainland or being born and raised on the mainland, also has been noted in the literature (Sanchez-Ayendez 1988; Canino and Canino 1993:481). These traditional gender roles have been discussed in association with machismo, which involves a belief that the male is traditionally responsible for the welfare and honor of the family, responsible for being the main provider for and protector of his family (Sanchez-Ayendez 1988; Ramirez 1992; Canino and Canino 1993); and marianismo, which involves a belief that "women are spiritually superior to men and, therefore, are capable of enduring suffering better than are men" (Canino and Canino 1993:481).

Considerable anthropological and social scientific research on Puerto Ricans on the island has been conducted by Puerto Rican social scientists and others (Steward et al. 1956; Mintz 1975; Buitrago-Ortiz et al. 1981; Seda-Bonilla 1964, 1970; Buitrago 1966, 1970; Duany 1988-89; Ramirez 1973, 1992; Burgos and Diaz Perez 1986; Marin and Triandis 1985; Koss-Chioino 1992; Koss 1980, 1987; Canino et al. 1987, 1990; Guarnaccia 1993.) These works address issues of social and cultural change in Puerto Rico, the existence and nature of Puerto Rican national identity, political and economic issues related to Puerto Rico's geopolitical status, gender issues, and mental health issues.

Although there has been considerable research on mental health issues among Puerto Ricans on the island, including studies of traditional Puerto Rican healers in mental health care (Koss-Chioino 1992; Koss 1980, 1987; Canino et al. 1987, 1990; Guarnaccia 1993), to my knowledge, few if any studies in Puerto Rico have focused on adaptation to chronic disabling diseases of a physical nature and, prior to the research described here, none have focused on chronic pain among island Puerto Ricans.

THE STUDY POPULATION

The Puerto Rican project is a study of chronic pain patients ($N = 100$) at an outpatient medical center near San Juan, Puerto Rico. The Puerto Rican project was reviewed and approved by the Human Subjects Review Committee at the State University of New York (SUNY) at Binghamton and by the director of the health center where the research occurred. Informed consent was obtained from each participant.

As at the New England Pain Control Center, all patients who participated in the Puerto Rican study were defined as having *chronic* pain using the guidelines set by the International Association for the Study of Pain (IASP) described in chapter 3. In the Puerto Rican study the same methods and procedures used at the New England center were employed: also, the same data were collected on each Puerto Rican patient so that comparisons could be made with the New England population. As with each of the New England ethnic groups, six Puerto Rican patients were selected for intensive case studies.

Most Puerto Rican patients were seen initially at the center (a few were not feeling well enough to come in, so first interviews were conducted in their homes), and follow-up interviews for intensive case studies were generally conducted in patients' homes. The six Puerto Rican case-study patients were interviewed and visited during at least two research periods. All Puerto Rican formal case-study interviews were tape recorded with the participants' permission and later transcribed. Patients in Puerto Rico were interviewed using the Spanish versions of the questionnaires described in chapter 3.

Initially, at the Puerto Rican medical center, which (like the New England center) has more than 6,000 patient visits per year, the staff reviewed medical records and identified patients whose chronic pain fit within the three main diagnostic categories found in the New England population. Each of these patients was contacted and asked to participate in the study; over 80% of those contacted agreed.[1] During the spring and summer months, from 1990 through 1993, 105 patients were administered the Ethnicity and Pain Survey to determine whether they considered themselves, and were by heritage, Puerto Ricans. Five patients and their parents were not born in Puerto Rico and were excluded from the database, leaving the 100 participants who are reported on here.

Medical Characteristics. In the Puerto Rican population, the range for pain duration was 6 months to 420 months, with a mean of 287.The majority of patients fell into one of three diagnostic categories: low-back pain (mechanical, radicular, or postsurgical), arthritis (osteo or rheumatoid), or some type of neuropathy (neuritis, neuralgia, or other neuropathies): approximately 50% had a primary diagnosis of arthritis and over 40% had a primary diagnosis of back pain. The most common past treatments for pain were nerve blocks, steroid injections, physical therapy, and chiropractic. The most commonly used medication classes were nonopiate analgesics, opiate analgesics, antidepressants, nonsteroid and steroid anti-inflammatories, and muscle relaxants.

Locus of Control Style Characteristics. A locus-of-control (LOC) mean was determined for the Puerto Rican population. Following the practice described by Krause and Stryker (1984), internal and external LOC groups were categorized by splitting the LOC scores at the study population's (made up of the 100 Puerto Ricans) mean. Those above the mean fell into the external group and those at and below the mean fell into the internal group. In the native Puerto Rican group, the majority of members fell into the *external* style (60%).

---

1. In Puerto Rico, those who refused to participate generally said they did not feel well enough to engage in an interview or did not want to travel to the medical center for the initial interview (and were not willing to have us conduct the initial visit in their homes). However, many of the Puerto Rican patients who agreed to participate also had severe arthritis or back pain, and the staff told us we had interviewed the majority of their most severe chronic pain patients as well as most of those with less severe pain and conditions. Therefore, physician-defined severity of condition does not appear to differentiate those who refused participation from those who agreed to participate. The medical or other center records on the patients who refused were not reviewed because to do so would have violated the informed consent standards and procedures of the project.

There were no significant relationships between the distribution of the two LOC styles and the other sociodemographic variables in this population, including age, gender, socioeconomic status (SES), and religion.

Sociodemographic Characteristics. The Puerto Rican population had an age mean of sixty years, and was 67% female. In Puerto Rico approximately 25% of subjects were receiving workers' compensation benefits. The Puerto Rican population had an education mean of approximately twelve years of education or the equivalent of a high school education. Household income levels were mainly in the working-class to middle-class range (over $7,000 up to $28,000), and the largest percentage of Puerto Rican subjects belonged to the semiskilled and skilled occupational categories. Catholics (88%) significantly outnumbered Protestants.

INTRA-PUERTO RICAN-GROUP VARIATION IN THE CHRONIC PAIN EXPERIENCE

Quantitative Analysis

In regard to pain *intensity*, in the analyses of variance (ANOVAs) there were only three variables that related to significant differences within the native Puerto Rican group; these were LOC style, age, and SES. The group with an external LOC style had a McGill Pain Questionnaire Pain Rating Index Total (MPQ-PRIT) intensity mean of 47, while the internal group's mean was significantly lower at 42 (table 6.1).

There were only 2 patients under age 40 in the Puerto Rican population, so only two age groups were compared. The older age group (61 and up) reported a significantly lower intensity mean on the MPQ-PRIT than did the younger age group consisting of those between 40 and 60 years of age. Regarding SES, those with higher levels of education and income reported significantly lower degrees of pain intensity on the MPQ-PRIT (table 6.1).

There also were significant differences in pain *responses* related to LOC style, heritage consistency, education and income, age, workers' compensation status, social support, and gender within the Puerto Rican population.

In behavioral responses, LOC style was related to several significant intragroup differences. First, in degree of expressiveness of pain, the internal LOC group reported less expressiveness of pain, with a mean of 11.9 out of 16, than the external group, with a mean of 14.9. Secondly, the external LOC style group reported significantly higher degrees of having to stop normal work inside and outside the home. The external LOC group also had significantly higher means for total interference in daily

Table 6.1. Significant Intra–Puerto Rican–Group Variations in Pain Intensity (MPQ-PRIT) by LOC Style, Age, and SES

| | LOC Style | | | | F-Ratio |
| | INTERNAL | | EXTERNAL | | |
	Mean	SD	Mean	SD	
Pain Intensity MPQ-PRIT	41.7	15.1	46.5	10.7	3.40*

| | AGE GROUPS | | | | F-ratio |
| | Ages 40–60 | | Ages 61 and up | | |
	Mean	SD	Mean	SD	
Pain Intensity MPQ-PRIT	50.2	10.1	38.5	12.7	26.20*

| | EDUCATION LEVEL | | | | | | | | F-ratio |
| | Under 12 Years | | High School Graduate | | Some College | | College Degree | | |
	Mean	SD	Mean	SD	Mean	SD	Mean	SD	
Pain Intensity MPQ-PRIT	51.2	8.2	44.8	13.2	43.1	14.1	39.8	12.9	4.40*

| | INCOME LEVELS | | | | | | F-ratio |
| | Under $7,000 | | $7,001–18,000 | | $18,001-up | | |
	Mean	SD	Mean	SD	Mean	SD	
Pain Intensity MPQ-PRIT	50.6	7.0	45.4	11.7	39.6	15.1	6.14*

SD = Standard Deviation
* $p < .01$

Table 6.2. Intra–Puerto Rican–Group Variations in Pain Responses by LOC Style

| Response Area | Internal LOC Style | | External LOC Style | | |
	Mean	SD	Mean	SD	F-Ratio
Expressiveness	11.9	3.6	14.9	4.4	12.89**
Work stoppage	4.1	1.6	5.2	1.5	12.20**
Total Interference in daily activities[b]	26.8	7.7	31.3	6.0	11.20**
Interference with Social Activities	2.4	1.1	3.1	.9	9.52*
Keeps Busy	2.9	1.3	2.3	1.2	6.56**
Degree of Depression	2.8	1.2	3.7	.8	18.87**
Degree of Worry	6.0	3.1	7.7	3.0	7.54**
Degree of Tension	3.1	1.3	3.8	.6	14.71**
Degree of Fear	1.5	1.1	2.4	1.3	13.92**
Pain = Unhappiness	1.7	1.2	2.7	1.3	15.83**
Can overcome pain[a]	3.7	.6	3.1	1.0	11.02**

Self-Defined Health Status[b] % of Group	Healthy 58%	Unhealthy/ Disabled 42%	Healthy 8%	Unhealthy/ Disabled 92%	Chi-square 8.12**

SD = Standard Deviation
*$p < .05$
**$p < .01$
[a]Higher score indicates belief one can overcome pain
[b]Patient asked to define self as healthy (H) or unhealthy/disabled (U/D).

activities and for interference with social activities. Members of the external group also were significantly less likely to report being able to find activities which kept them busy and active than were internal group members (table 6.2).

LOC style also was related to significant intragroup variations in emotional response to pain, with the areas showing significant differences being degrees of self-reported depression, fear, tension, and worry—in each case the internal style group had a significantly lower mean (table 6.2).

In several attitudinal areas there were significant LOC differences as well: those who had an external LOC style reported a statistically significant higher level of agreement that as long as they had pain they would never have a happy and fulfilling life, while those in the internal group expressed disagreement with that statement. Belief in the ability to overcome the pain also was related to LOC style in Puerto Ricans: members of the internal group were significantly more likely to agree that they were determined to overcome the pain than were members of the external group. Finally, there was a significant difference in self-defined health status between the two LOC style groups. In the internal LOC group, 58% defined themselves as healthy, compared to only 8% of the external group (table 6.2).

As in the New England population, a sense of control had a significant impact on the chronic pain experiences of native Puerto Ricans. Those Puerto Ricans with a sense of internal control over their life circumstances were adapting to their pain experiences in a more positive manner as they were experiencing less interference with daily activities and lower degrees of depression, worry, tension, fear, and unhappiness; and, despite the chronic pain, they were more apt to define themselves as healthy and to agree that they could overcome the pain.

Age was related to significant differences in several response areas, including work stoppage; degree of expression; levels of worry, anger, and depression; patients' abilities to keep busy and active; and views on pain and happiness (table 6.3). In each case the oldest age group was coping better and reporting less work stoppage and less worry, anger, depression, and unhappiness than the younger age group. The actual means for each response are provided in table 6.3. This pattern is similar to the relationship between age and pain response variations at the New England center, where the oldest age group also was generally adapting more effectively to the pain experience than younger age groups.

Among island Puerto Ricans, high heritage consistency correlated less with a belief that pain meant a life of unhappiness and unfulfillment (table 6.4). In other words, stronger ties to the cultural group and a lifestyle reflective of one's traditional culture lessened the belief that throughout the duration of pain one would never have a happy and fulfilling life. Among native Puerto Ricans, high heritage consistency also correlated with a stronger belief that one could overcome pain and with higher degrees of reported support from family and friends. Finally, as heritage consistency rose, degrees of tension, anger, and fear went down (table 6.4).

Reports of support from family and friends during the pain episode, and reports that despite the pain, the patient was able to find activities that kept him or her busy and active, indicated that as the degree of support went up, so did the ability to keep busy. Degree of social support from family and friends also was correlated with significant differences in work stoppage: as social support went up, degree of having to stop normal work went down (table 6.4).

Table 6.3. Intra–Puerto Rican–Group Variations in Pain Responses by Age

| | Age Groups | | | | |
| | Ages 40–60 | | Ages 61 and up | | |
	Mean	SD	Mean	SD	F-Ratio
Work Stoppage	5.1	1.6	4.4	1.6	3.95*
Degree of Expression	14.7	3.9	12.6	4.6	5.70*
Keeps Busy	2.2	1.3	2.9	1.2	7.57**
Degree of Worries	7.7	3.1	6.3	3.1	5.01*
Degree of Anger	2.9	1.2	2.3	1.4	5.33*
Degree of Depression	3.6	.8	3.0	1.3	8.76**
Pain = Unhappiness	2.8	1.3	1.9	1.3	5.55*

SD = Standard Deviation
*$p < .05$
**$p < .01$

The findings that Puerto Ricans with high degrees of heritage consistency and of social support are coping better than those with low heritage consistency and social support reflect the Puerto Rican view of the family as the paramount mediating institution between the individual and his or her social and physical reality (Sanchez-Ayendez 1984, 1988). In this orientation, the idea that individuals are not capable of doing everything and, therefore, should rely on others for assistance underlies interdependent family relations (Bastida 1979:70–71).

SES correlated with two response differences among Puerto Ricans (tables 6.4 and 6.5). Higher education levels correlated with less agreement that as long as one had pain one would have an unhappy and unfulfilled life (table 6.4). Education also correlated with seeking a reason for pain. The higher the education level, the less likely one was to still be seeking a reason for the pain (table 6.4). This may occur because those with a higher education level (which was often also associated with a higher household income level) were more likely to have had a history of aggressively seeking medical evaluations (including trips to the mainland for consultation and treatment in several cases) and thus may have attained a satisfactory explanation for their pain.

In addition, those with a college education were less expressive about their pain, reported less work stoppage, and had less pain-related worry and depression than those with less education. Those with a college degree also were less likely to agree that continued pain meant they would never have a fulfilling and happy life (table 6.5).

Table 6.4. Intra–Puerto Rican–Group Correlations

	Pearson Correlation Coefficients
Heritage Consistency and	
Pain = Unhappiness	−.31*
Ability to Overcome Pain	.32*
Degree of Family and Friends' Support	.27*
Degree of Tension	−.25*
Degree of Anger	−.21**
Degree of Fear	−.35*
Education and	
Pain = Unhappiness	−.29*
Seeks Reason for Pain	−.30*
Degree of Family and Friends' Support and	
Ability to Keep Busy and Active	.28*
Degree of Work Stoppage	−.25*

*$p < .05$
**$p < .01$

Income was also related to significant response differences: again, those with higher incomes reported less severe work stoppage and emotional responses and were less likely to agree that continued pain meant continued unhappiness (table 6.5). (The pattern for differences in responses related to occupational status was almost identical to that for income and education and thus will not be presented here.)

As in several New England center ethnic groups, sufficient economic resources (which were generally associated with higher education levels and professional occupational status) appear to lessen the stress of the chronic pain experience among native Puerto Ricans.

Workers' compensation status was also related to several intragroup response differences (table 6.6). First, those on compensation reported significantly higher levels of work stoppage (inside and outside the home) than did non–workers' compensation subjects. Those receiving workers' compensation were significantly less likely to agree that they could overcome their pain. These workers' compensation relationships also are similar to those found at the New England center and described in chapter 5.

In Puerto Rico, gender was associated with significant differences in three quantitative variables. Women were more likely than men to still be seeking a reason for their pain, while men were more likely to report they did not believe in taking pain medications. While both men and women had high means for tension, the female group, with a mean of 3.7,

Table 6.5. Intra–Puerto Rican–Group Variations in Pain Responses by SES

EDUCATION LEVEL

RESPONSE	Under 12 Years		High School Graduate		Some College		College Degree		F-Ratio
	Mean	SD	Mean	SD	Mean	SD	Mean	SD	
Degree of Expression	16.5	3.4	13.2	3.8	14.0	4.2	11.4	4.4	8.14**
Work Stoppage	5.1	1.5	5.1	1.7	5.2	1.2	3.9	1.7	4.58**
Degree of Worries	8.5	2.9	7.2	2.9	6.8	3.1	5.9	3.1	3.65**
Degree of Depression	3.8	.6	3.5	1.0	3.3	1.1	2.9	1.4	3.13*
Pain = Unhappiness	3.0	1.2	2.1	1.3	2.1	1.4	1.8	1.2	4.68*

INCOME LEVELS

	Under $7,000		$7,001–18,000		$18,001-up		F-Ratio
	Mean	SD	Mean	SD	Mean	SD	
Work Stoppage	5.0	1.7	5.3	1.2	4.1	1.7	6.60**
Degree of Expression	14.5	3.2	15.4	4.3	11.5	4.2	9.39**
Degree of Worries	6.9	2.6	8.0	3.2	6.2	3.2	3.40*
Degree of Tension	3.7	.7	3.8	.6	3.1	1.3	6.70**

(Continued on next page)

Table 6.5. (*Cont'd.*)

	INCOME LEVELS						
	Under $7,000		$7,001–18,000		$18,001-up		
	Mean	SD	Mean	SD	Mean	SD	F-Ratio
Degree of Depression	3.7	.6	3.6	.9	2.7	1.4	8.19**
Pain = Unhappiness	2.6	1.4	2.5	1.3	1.8	1.2	4.30*

SD = Standard Deviation
$p < .05$
**$p < .01$

Table 6.6. Significant Intra–Puerto Rican–Group Variations in Pain Responses by Workers' Compensation and Gender

| | Variation by Workers' Compensation Status | | | | |
| | Receiving Compensation | | No Compensation | | |
	Mean	SD	Mean	SD	F-Ratio
Work Stoppage	5.4	1.5	4.6	1.6	5.17*
Belief that One Can Overcome Pain[a]	3.1	1.1	3.5	.8	3.71*

| | Variation by Gender | | | | |
| | Male | | Female | | |
	Mean	SD	Mean	SD	F-Ratio
Believes in Taking Pain Medication	1.9	1.3	1.2	.8	5.11*
Seeks Reason for Pain	.9	1.0	1.9	1.7	4.21*
Degree of Tension	3.2	1.3	3.7	.8	6.89**

SD = Standard Deviation
*$p < .05$
**$p < .01$
[a]Higher score indicates belief one can overcome pain.

reported a significantly higher degree of tension associated with the pain than did the male group, which had a mean of 3.2 (table 6.6).

Qualitative Analysis

On a qualitative level, differences in response to pain related to gender and to employment status were evident among Puerto Ricans. Men who had ceased employment appeared to cope less well than men who were still employed and than women generally (regardless of employment status). Many men who could no longer work, such as Jesus described in chapter 1, reported a great loss of self-esteem and increased depression, and several reported having attempted or seriously considered suicide. (The chief physician at the medical center in Puerto Rico confirmed suicide attempts by several of the male patients.) In contrast, none of the women in the Puerto Rican sample reported attempts or consideration of suicide; in addition, those Puerto Rican men who remained employed (such as Manuel described in chapter 1) did not report suicidal tendencies.

Culturally specific gender-role expectations are probably among the factors influencing the gender differences in response to the chronic pain experience, as overall in the Puerto Rican study group there was no significant difference in diagnosis or severity of condition between males and females. Among Puerto Ricans on the island (and on the mainland), the definition of "maleness" refers to a man's ability to be a good provider for his family and to his ability to control his emotions and be self-sufficient, not only, as noted in chapter 4, to often-cited negative aspects of machismo (Sanchez-Ayendez 1984:243; Ramirez 1992).

Puerto Rican women also reported that two of the most distressful aspects of having chronic pain were related to gender-role expectations— providing social support to family and friends and keeping a clean household. However, while noting that pain interfered with meeting these obligations, the majority of Puerto Rican women reported finding ways to fulfill them. Several women, I learned, had devised new ways to do household chores; for example, one woman with back problems said she lies on the floor on her stomach in order to dust and clean under the beds because she cannot bend over to do so. Other women told of meeting social obligations in new ways, including increased reliance on phone conversations to provide social support to family and friends rather than in-person visits. Thus, overall, the majority of Puerto Rican women reported devising strategies for meeting major obligations despite the chronic pain.

Another qualitative theme within the Puerto Rican group was a marked tendency to express pain verbally and behaviorally, as both genders winced, groaned, grimaced, and emotionally described their pain in a very open manner. Even Puerto Ricans who were adapting to their pain experiences quite effectively and who thought they had a happy life considered it appropriate to express pain openly.

Several case studies from the Puerto Rican population further illustrate both cultural patterning of the pain experience and intragroup variations as well.

PUERTO RICAN CASE STUDIES

A case study of a native Puerto Rican woman, Maria, interviewed in 1990 and 1993, demonstrates the Puerto Rican tendency, which cut across all socioeconomic classes, to be expressive about pain. Maria's case study also shows how possessing an attitude of self-control can mediate the chronic pain experience.

Similar to Manuel described in chapter 1, Maria has a sense of control and a self-proclaimed ability to cope effectively with the chronic pain associated with rheumatoid arthritis. She is a Puerto Rican widow in her mid-seventies who now belongs to the Puerto Rican upper-middle class.

Maria was raised on a plantation, one of ten children of poor plantation workers. Her mother was determined to educate her children but, due to poverty, Maria often lacked shoes and her mother refused to endure the shame of her daughter attending grammar school without shoes. During those periods, as the family saved money for shoes, Maria taught herself. She said, "I was a fighter, I took my older brothers' books and read them." Poverty also ruled out attending high school. This made her "very angry and frustrated," and eventually her parents sent her to commercial classes. She said, "But I wanted science and I continued to fight to attend high school. My best friend was allowed to go and I envied her so much. . . . This was a black period in my life."

However, she never gave up her dream. She married her first husband when she was in her late teens and soon thereafter had a son. She reported repeated physical and psychological abuse by her first husband. Nonetheless, while married to him, Maria finally was able to attend and finish high school—over her husband's strenuous objections and despite repeated beatings. During that period Maria had to hide her schoolbooks from her husband and study by flashlight after he had gone to sleep to avoid his anger. With great determination, she struggled to leave this first marriage and continue her education. Living in extreme poverty at the time, she managed to overcome many obstacles to obtain a divorce and complete undergraduate and graduate degrees while caring for her son. Maria said, "I was determined and fighting to get that degree." She succeeded and became a health professional. Later she married another health professional and she said this thirty-year marriage was a wonderful partnership full of love and caring. After completing her advanced degree, Maria worked in a health-care field until semiretirement about five years ago. She still engages in consultations and volunteer activities.

Maria has suffered from rheumatoid arthritis for more than thirty years. As a health professional, she has in-depth knowledge of her disease, and also expressed the belief that the many beatings she endured from her first husband may in some way have contributed to the development of her arthritis. The joints of Maria's hands and feet are badly deformed from the arthritis, and she also has arthritis of the spine.

She said that she has some control over her pain much of the time, and scored in the internal range on the LOC questions. In addition, her life history suggests that, despite often overwhelming odds, Maria has almost always exhibited a sense of purpose and control and has been able to exert substantial influence over the direction of her life.

When she first learned of her disease, Maria studied the literature on it and devised a daily exercise program which she has consistently maintained for thirty years and to which she attributes her ability to remain active. She also uses a variety of helpful devices in her home, such as special handles on the faucets and special rails in the shower. Maria reported that the treatments provided by her physician at the center (which often involved steroid injections into especially painful joints) provide some temporary pain relief—although she is never pain free.

Maria described severe pain episodes in which she would lie on the floor screaming and beating her fists against the floor in open expression of her pain. Despite her expressiveness, Maria nonetheless saw herself as in control of her pain and her life. She said she believes a positive attitude and a lot of determination, as well as her daily exercise routine, has enabled her to live with a serious and painful disease for more than thirty years and still have a good life. She remains interested in helping others and believes she still has a lot to offer.

The next Puerto Rican case study involves Carlos, a skilled tradesman with a high-school education, married with two grown children. Carlos's response to his chronic pain and associated disability is much less positive than Maria's, even though his medical conditions are substantially less severe than hers. He has low-back pain from degenerative disk disease and degenerative joint disease of the spine. Sixty-two years-old, he has had chronic pain in his back since a 1978 accident at work. He did, however, continue to work for four years after the accident, and during that time he advanced to supervisor. When in 1982 the pain became more severe and he could no longer fulfill his work obligations, Carlos had to leave work on Social Security Disability. (He did not receive workers' compensation because his back condition in 1982 could not be directly attributed to his work accident in 1978.) He retired permanently in 1985. He currently receives Social Security benefits that are substantially less than his former salary. Since 1982, he has had several spinal surgeries, including removal of disks in his lower back and a fusion of cervical vertebrae.

Carlos displayed considerable pain behavior during interviews. On several occasions he had to stand because of back pain and associated leg pain. He expressed concern about having to cease employment and about the loss of a decent salary. Carlos also said he worries a lot about his Social Security benefits and believes that the meager benefits may actually decline in the future, "due to the fickleness of the [U.S.] bureaucracy."

Carlos reported severe interference with social activities, driving, walking, and sleeping, and expressed great dissatisfaction with his inability to do repairs and other household chores. He sees a psychologist once a month for depression primarily associated with, he said, "my lack of usefulness." He also was once a "top-notch" social dancer who won numerous trophies. But he is no longer able to dance, his favorite pastime, and he expressed distress over this loss.

Carlos is a very proud man who refuses to use the cane which has been prescribed in public, even though he admits it provides minor relief when he uses it at home. He has been told he faces future surgeries for removal of spurs from his fused cervical vertebrae and for removal of meniscus and cartilage from both knees. He is very worried about these surgeries and said his greatest fear is that he will become completely incapacitated.

As with other Puerto Rican men who have had to cease employment due to their pain (such as Jesus described in chapter 1), Carlos's sense of self worth has been severely affected by having to stop work. He is also extremely distressed by his current economic situation and expressed great fear for his economic future. In addition, he said he worries about his wife, who has always been a full-time housewife. He fears he will die and she will be left alone without sufficient income and resources.

Carlos currently agrees strongly that as long as he has pain, he will never have a fulfilling and happy life. He believes he had substantial control over the direction of his life prior to having to cease work, and he cites his promotion to supervisor as an example of how, despite the pain he was experiencing at the time, his own hard work led to improvements in his lifestyle. However, Carlos said that much of the time now he feels he does not have control over the direction of his life and that he has almost no influence over the things that happen to him.

Clearly it is not the pain *per se* that has led to his current sense of having no control over his life circumstances. From 1978 to 1982, Carlos continued to work and won a promotion—he said he felt in control of his life during that period even though he regularly experienced substantial amounts of back pain. According to Carlos, he lost that sense of control when the pain became so severe in 1982 that he could no longer carry out his duties and was forced to go on disability. Carlos said that not being able to work and earn a decent living is what led to the loss of control. As a result of having to cease employment, he reported high degrees of anger, tension, and fear, and he now defines his health status as disabled.

As with Jesus and other Puerto Rican men who had to stop work, Carlos ties his sense of manhood, self-esteem, and self-control to his ability to work and be a good provider for his family. For these Puerto Rican men, loss of employment capabilities has led to loss of self-esteem, manliness, and control. Even Manuel (whose case was presented in chapter 1), who is doing well and is still employed, commented that he can cope with pain and chronic disease precisely because he can still engage in the work he so values.

Of course, a similar pattern was found among the New England Latino men. This same pattern was evident in case studies of two Puerto

Rican immigrants to New England—Juan's case, discussed in chapter 4, and Ricardo's, discussed in chapter 5.

In sharp contrast to Carlos's experience with chronic pain is that of Sonia Rodriguez, a Puerto Rican woman in her late forties who has a severe case of rheumatoid arthritis which began in 1963 when she was twenty years old. (Sonia's real name is used here at her explicit request.) Sonia's family history includes both parents and one sister with osteo-arthritis and a paternal grandmother with rheumatoid arthritis from whom Sonia believes she inherited the disease. Sonia also has had severe stomach problems, including bleeding ulcers, related to various anti-inflammatory medications she has taken for arthritis. She takes opiates for relief when the pain is especially severe, has occasional steroid injections into especially painful joints, and takes various anti-ulcer medications.

Sonia is a remarkable woman. The first time we met in 1992, she arrived at the center for our interview in an ambulance. The staff who arranged the interview said Sonia was unable to walk because she had to have her artificial hip joint removed due to severe infection. Thus she was transported by ambulance, declining an offer for us to come to her. She enjoys getting out.

Expecting to meet a woman who was very ill and handicapped, Sonia proved to be a surprise. She is a beautiful, well-dressed, and well-groomed woman who smiles often, laughs often, and has a wonderful sense of humor. Joking and laughing with the ambulance attendants as they brought her into the office, it was soon apparent that Sonia had a risque sense of humor. She said she especially enjoys outings with friends to male exotic-dance shows and that her favorite entertainers are the Chippendales (a male exotic-dance team).

Sonia's hands and feet are badly deformed from the arthritis, and she has now been without a joint in one hip for over three years. She is con-fined mainly to a wheelchair, although with the use of an elevated shoe and a walker she manages to walk for short distances within her home with difficulty (but wants to continue since it gives her a sense of indepen-dence which she cherishes).

In addition to arthritis, Sonia has severe osteoporosis, for which she now gives herself prescribed calcium injections. This condition makes another attempt at hip surgery questionable, but she continues to hope that one day soon she will be able to have a successful hip replacement.

With a high-school education and some post-high-school secretarial and accounting courses, despite her severe case of rheumatoid arthritis, Sonia worked for twenty-five years until 1988, when she fell in the shower, broke her hip, and could no longer walk. She first worked as a secretary and later, at the same firm, the owner moved her into a receptionist position when her hands became too deformed to type—the firm did not want to lose her and was willing to make this work reassignment. Her former employer still values her highly and calls her often (she reported that he tells others in the office, "You can't replace a Sonia"). Given her obvious intelligence, outgoing personality, and cheerfulness, it is not hard to imagine that Sonia is missed by those she worked with, and she maintains close ties, by phone and in person, with her former employer and fellow workers.

Before she lost her ability to walk, Sonia lived alone and had a very active social life. She dated frequently and especially loved to go dancing. Never married, Sonia moved in with her parents after breaking her hip in 1988 and still lives with them. She is also very close to her sisters, nieces, and nephews. One sister, who is a nurse, is especially helpful, and one niece spends a great deal of time with her, often taking her for outings in her wheelchair. Sonia believes her family is one of the main reasons she still feels a sense of purpose and worth—she said: "They need me and come to me for emotional help. If they see me down, it demoralizes the family. So I know I am needed."

Sonia reported experiencing severe depression following her initial fall and associated broken hip, and another severe depression and loss of faith in God when the infected artificial joint had to be removed. But she said she gradually regained her faith. She saw a psychologist briefly during both of those episodes, but she credits her sister with pulling her out of her depressions and insisting that Sonia must not lose her faith in God. Sonia said she now does not dwell on what she can no longer have or do, but rather focuses on the good things she does have in her life, including her family and many good friends. Sonia said a person has to "live with the life they are dealt." She said she has a good life and that she is in control of her pain during much of the time. She also expressed a belief that doctors will someday find a cure for rheumatoid arthritis—hopefully within her lifetime.

Her "strong character," her faith in God, her doctor at the center, and her family all help her to cope with her pain and disability, Sonia said. She has been seeing the same center physician since 1969 and they have a close and supportive relationship. In addition, the other staff members and several other patients there are very fond of Sonia and provide substantial psychosocial support and social contact.

Sonia said she spends a great deal of time each day on the phone with friends and relatives—she estimates she engages in a minimum of eight phone conversations per day. The phone has become her major form of social interaction since her mobility became very limited. She also loves to watch television and said her evenings are filled with pleasure because of the many good evening shows. Despite the severe pain she often suffers, and her disability, Sonia said she tries very hard to "dominate the pain." She said she will not give up, will keep going, and will continue to try to enjoy life.

Despite her positive attitude and deliberate attempts to focus on good things, Sonia admits she has days when the pain is extremely severe, during which time she tends to withdraw into herself, preferring to be alone. On those days, which she calls "being in crisis" (this phrase was used by numerous Puerto Rican patients to describe their bad spells), Sonia said she cries and often moans and groans in pain.

Sonia receives a small income from Social Security Disability Insurance, but with her many prescription medications and medical bills, she has substantial financial concerns. A recent attempt on her part to switch to generic drugs to save money resulted, in her view, in a "crisis." She has therefore had to go back to brand-name drugs despite their higher cost.

Overall, Sonia has one of the most severe cases of arthritis encountered in either study. By biomedical standards she is a very ill woman with severe disabilities. Yet Sonia exemplifies the study finding that type or severity of disease often has no relationship to patients' responses to pain and illness. Sonia is one of the most optimistic, positive, and cheerful people I have ever met. She said she is determined to overcome the pain and very strongly disagrees with the statement "As long as I am in pain, I will never have a fulfilling and happy life." When asked to define her health status, she said, "in between healthy and unhealthy. I need some help, so I guess I am somewhat disabled. But I am glad to be alive. There are many people in the world who are much worse off than I am."

CHAPTER 7

COMPARISONS OF PUERTO RICANS
WITH NEW ENGLAND LATINOS
AND ANGLO AMERICANS

A COMPARISON OF NEW ENGLAND LATINOS
AND ISLAND PUERTO RICANS

How does the island Puerto Rican chronic pain experience compare over-all with the chronic pain experiences of the New England Latino popula-tion, the majority of which consisted of Puerto Rican immigrants to the mainland? A comparison of the experiences of the two Latino groups illustrates cultural influences on the chronic pain experience as well as the impact of the migration experience.

Because the vast majority of the New England sample had back pain and few had arthritis or fell into the neuropathy category, I will compare the New England Latinos (N = 44) to a similar subgroup from the larger Puerto Rican population, consisting of those who have a main diagnosis of back pain (N = 48).

Although the native Puerto Rican back-pain group had more females in it than in the New England Latino group, the difference in gender dis-tributions between the two was not statistically significant. There was a significant difference in mean education levels between the two groups, as the New England Latinos had an education mean of 9 years while the native back-pain Puerto Rican subgroup's education mean was 12 years. There also was a significant difference between the two groups in mean age; the mean of 59 years for the back pain Puerto Rican subgroup was significantly higher than the New England Latinos mean of 41 (table 7.1).

There was a significant difference in pain duration between the two Latino groups: the New England Latino group had a pain duration mean of 54 months, while the back pain Puerto Rican subgroup had a duration mean of 236 months (table 7.1). Two major factors explain the duration difference. First, the native Puerto Rican population was older and, therefore, in relation to their chronic conditions, would be expected to have experienced a longer period of pain. Secondly, the Puerto Rican medical center has been in operation for more than thirty years, and many of the subjects have been patients for that entire period. In contrast, the New England center was established as recently as 1976, and only a few Latino patients have been coming to the center for more than three years. However, the age of onset of chronic pain does not appear to differ between the New England population and Puerto Rican population. Most island Puerto Ricans began to have chronic back pain while in their thirties or forties, which is also the age of onset in the majority of New England Latino patients.

No statistically significant difference was found in the distributions of the two locus-of-control (LOC) styles between these two Latino back-pain groups (chi-square = .21, p = .64). In both Latino back-pain groups, those in the external LOC group outnumbered those in the internal group. There also were no significant differences between the two Latino groups in types of current pain medications or in types of past treatments for the pain.

In the combined study population (made up of the 44 New England Latinos and the 48 back-pain Puerto Ricans), there was a significant difference in reported *pain intensity* between the Puerto Rican subgroup and the New England Latino group. Using the MPQ-PRIT intensity mean, the native Puerto Rican subgroup had a higher mean of 46, while the New England Latino group's mean was 41 (table 7.2). This difference between the two Latino groups remained in regression analysis when other variables were controlled (see table F.5 in appendix F for Regression).

Based on the qualitative data, I hypothesize that one of the factors in the lower *reported intensity* in the New England Latino group is the different cultural context in which they seek care and treatment. It is very possible that the New England Latinos have reported less pain intensity as a response to the dominance of Anglo American attitudes among the New England center's staff, which then leads to rewards (positive attention and praise) for stoicism and nonexpressiveness of pain and, in effect (but probably unconsciously), punishments for expressing pain through lack of positive attention and negative facial and verbal expressions. As New England Latinos must seek care in such a different cultural setting from their native Puerto Rico (where both patients and health-care providers shared the attitude that expressiveness of pain was both acceptable and entirely appropriate), they probably are gradually assimilating to the Anglo American practices of nonexpressiveness and less reporting of

Table 7.1. Significant Differences in Characteristics of Two Latino Groups

Characteristic	New England Latinos	Island Back-Pain Puerto Ricans	F-Ratio	P
Education[a]				
Mean	8.7	12.4	27.50	.00
SD	3.4	3.7		
Age				
Mean	41.2	59.4	63.36	.00
SD	10.5	11.1		
Pain Duration[b]				
Mean	54.1	236.2	93.2	.00
SD	56.0	111.7		

SD = Standard Deviation
[a]Education recorded in number of years of education.
[b]Pain duration recorded in number of months in pain.

pain—at least within the medical setting. Although compared to Anglo Americans they were still considered very expressive, they were probably less so than they would have been in a Puerto Rican health-care setting, where expressiveness meets with no disapproval. This explanation seems plausible since among New England Latinos, as generation level rose, degree of expressiveness of pain went down.

In regression analysis, which controlled for the differences in age, pain duration, and education between the two Latino groups, there were *no* significant differences between the two in any *behavioral responses*, including work stoppage, interference in daily activities, or expressiveness of the pain. This finding of no differences in expressiveness does not contradict the hypothesis offered above concerning reports of pain intensity, as the majority of questions concerning expressiveness relate to expressiveness in family and social settings rather than the medical setting.

In regard to *psychological/emotional responses*, the regression analyses showed no significant differences in degree of tension, depression, unhappiness, or worry between the two Latino groups. The New England Latinos did report a significantly higher degree of anger (table 7.2) associated with their pain (mean of 3.7 out of 4), than the native Puerto Rican subgroup's mean of 2.5 (see appendix F, table F.6 for the regression table).

In *attitudinal responses* there were no significant differences in attitudes towards pain and unhappiness or the state of one's health between the two Latino groups. Both the New England Latinos and native back-pain Puerto Rican groups had a high percentage of members who categorized their health as unhealthy/disabled. Also, there were no differences

Table 7.2. Significant Differences in Pain Intensity and Responses between the Two Latino Groups

	New England Latinos	Island Back-Pain Puerto Ricans	F-Ratio	p
MPQ-PRIT Intensity				
Mean	40.6	46.4		
SD	13.5	12.0	4.48	.04*
Anger				
Mean[a]	3.7	2.5		
SD	.8	1.4	16.85	.00**

SD = Standard Deviation
[a]Pain-related degree of anger; higher scores indicates greater degree of anger.
*$p < .05$
**$p < .01$

between the two Latino groups in reported social support from family and friends during the pain experience, and no differences in the degree to which patients sought and used the advice of family and friends regarding treatment of their pain and disease. In both areas, both Latino groups had high means, indicating they sought and used advice of family and friends often and that they received high degrees of social support.

Within the combined study population (consisting in this case of only the back-pain Puerto Ricans and the New England Latinos), the quantitative analyses revealed that gender was not related to significant differences in pain *intensity*. However, gender was related to significant differences in degree of pain-related anger (see table 7.3 for actual anger means). In addition, the female group's mean for finding activities to keep themselves busy and active despite the pain was significantly higher than the male group's mean—indicating that women were able to find activities that kept them busy and active despite the pain, while men were not able to do so (table 7.3). Gender was the only variable related to significant differences in keeping busy in the combined Latino population. These findings of gender differences in the combined Latino population support the qualitative data, which consistently showed Latino women to be coping better with the pain experience than Latino men.

Education was the only variable in the analyses of variance (ANOVAs) (or the regression) that was related to significant differences in work stoppage in the combined Latino back-pain study population—the higher the education level, the lower the work stoppage (table 7.3).

In summary, the statistical analyses showed that the variables most often associated with significant differences in pain responses in the combined Latino population were age, LOC style, gender and education.

Table 7.3. Significant Gender and Education Differences in Pain Responses in
Combined Latino Back-Pain Population

| RESPONSE AREA | GENDER DIFFERENCES | | |
	FEMALES	MALES	F-ratio
Anger[a]			
Mean	2.6	3.5	
SD	1.3	1.1	9.9**
Finds Activities[b]			
Mean	2.5	1.8	
SD	1.3	1.2	5.2*

| | EDUCATION DIFFERENCES | | | | |
	Under 12 Years	High School	Some College	College Degree	F-Ratio
Work Stoppage[a]					
Mean	6.7	6.5	5.4	4.5	
SD	1.6	1.9	1.1	1.7	7.34**

SD = Standard Deviation
*p < .05
**p < .01
[a]Pain-related anger or work stoppage; higher score means greater degree.
[b]Degree to which patients agree that they have been able to find activities which keep them
  busy and active despite the pain; higher score indicates greater agreement.

Summary of Comparison of Native Puerto Rican and New England Latino Back-Pain Patients

This quantitative comparison showed major similarities between the two
Latino groups in expressiveness of pain and other behavioral responses,
in emotional responses, and in attitudes toward the relationship between
chronic pain and both health status and happiness. These similarities
clearly relate to shared cultural norms, attitudes, beliefs, and standards.
Both Latino groups also had high means for seeking and using treatment
advice of family and friends and for receiving social support from family
and friends. These means reflect the Puerto Rican attitude that individuals
should rely on family members for assistance (Bastida 1979:70–71).

Although the New England Latino group had a higher percentage in
the external LOC style subgroup than did the native Puerto Rican subgroup, the difference was not statistically significant. The finding that
both Latino groups had a majority in the external-LOC-style group further supports the hypothesis (offered in chapter 3) that historical and current political, social, and economic conditions, as well as the Latin
American cultural orientation toward reality, help explain why the

majority of Latinos tend to believe that external factors control their life circumstances.

The difference in degree of pain-related anger between the two Latino groups was probably related to differences between them in socioeconomic status (SES) and to the stress of the migration experience among the New England Latinos. As discussed in chapter 5 and earlier in this chapter, the intra-cultural-group analyses among New England Latinos and among native Puerto Ricans showed a relationship between SES and variations in pain-related tension, worries, etc. In each case, the lower the SES level the higher the pain-related tension, worries, etc.

In fact, SES and migration stress are probably related in the case of the New England Latinos. As was often the case among the Puerto Rican immigrants to New England (such as Juan, who was discussed earlier), if a migrant with back pain had a high-school education or less and spoke little or no English, there were few non-manual-labor employment opportunities available on the mainland. Also, given that the migrant's wages were generally low, the workers' compensation benefits or disability income the migrant received were also quite low. This left the New England Latino back-pain patient with severe financial problems in addition to chronic pain.

Also, as numerous New England Latinos said (including Juan and Ricardo), they came to the mainland expressly to make a better living and future for themselves and their families; thus, the economic hardships of the chronic pain experience shattered dreams many immigrants had worked very hard to attain. It is not surprising under such circumstances that the New England Latinos experienced higher levels of anger than the native Puerto Ricans.

An additional migration-related factor affecting the New England Latinos' response to chronic pain was the cultural context of care on the mainland. For Latino patients not fluent in English, no psychological and occupational therapies were available because of the language barrier. In addition, initial psychological assessment instruments were not available in Spanish, so Latino patients who did not read English did not receive the assessment other New England patients received. Since there were also no interpreters available at the New England pain center for any purpose, New England Latinos who did not speak English often brought children with them to translate their concerns to physicians and nurses and to translate what providers said back to them. One can certainly see the potential for major problems with patient-provider communications under such conditions. It is no wonder the New England Latinos were angry and frustrated under such health-care conditions.

In summary, the comparison of back-pain Puerto Ricans and New England Latinos demonstrated many more similarities than differences in behavioral, attitudinal, and psychosocial responses to the pain experience. These many similarities appear to be related to shared cultural beliefs, attitudes, meanings, and norms for appropriate behaviors. The major significant psychosocial difference between the two groups was in anger associated with the pain. This difference probably related to differences in SES status and conditions of the migration experience, including the frustrations of dealing with a health-care system that had a different language and different cultural beliefs and values.

The difference in reported pain intensity between the New England Latino and the back-pain Puerto Rican groups was not attributable to differences in pain duration, as duration was controlled for in the regression and was not related to pain intensity at a statistically significant level. The intensity difference between the two groups remained significant when age (which was significantly related to the intensity variation) was controlled; therefore, the difference in age between the two Latino groups does not explain the intensity differences between them. The two Latino groups were similar diagnostically, so difference in medical condition was not the reason for the intensity variation. The difference in reported pain intensity, with the New England Latinos reporting less pain intensity than the native Puerto Ricans, was probably related to the cultural context of health care (different cultural standards for expression and reporting of pain) and thus also related to the New England Latinos' migration status.

ANGLO AMERICAN AND ISLAND PUERTO RICAN COMPARISON

A comparison of the chronic pain experiences of Anglo Americans and island Puerto Ricans will illustrate the difference between two cultural rather than ethnic groups—and will further assess the role of culture in the chronic pain experience without the effects of migration stress and without language-related communication problems with providers. Each of these cultural groups lives in a context where the health-care setting is dominated by their own cultural group.

There were significant differences between the 100 Anglo Americans and 100 Puerto Ricans in distribution of the three most common diagnostic categories; therefore, subgroups composed of those with the diagnosis of back pain (from each larger cultural group) will be compared. These two subgroups consist of the group of back-pain native Puerto Ricans (N = 48) and a comparable group of back-pain Anglo Americans (N = 48)—randomly selected from the larger group of Anglo Americans with back pain.

There were no significant differences in these two back-pain cultural groups in socioeconomic status (SES) as measured by income, occupation, and education; workers' compensation status; types of pain medication being taken; and types of past treatments and surgeries for the pain. While the Puerto Rican back-pain group had slightly more females in it than the Anglo American back-pain group, there was not a significant difference between the two in gender distributions.

As indicated in table 7.4, there was a significant difference in religion, with the majority of native Puerto Ricans being Catholic (89%), and over 50% of Anglo Americans being Protestant. The only other sociodemographic difference between the groups was in mean age. The age mean of the Puerto Ricans was 61 years, significantly higher than that of the Anglo Americans, which was 42 years. There was also a difference in pain duration means: the back-pain Puerto Rican group's duration mean was 227 months, and the back-pain Anglo American group's duration mean was 61 months.

There were no significant differences in LOC style distributions between the two back pain groups. Anglo Americans were somewhat less external (47% were external) than Puerto Ricans (58% were external), but the difference was not statistically significant for these two subgroups (chi-square = .028, p = .87).

Inter-Cultural-Group Pain Intensity Variation

In this combined back-pain population, made up of the island back-pain Puerto Ricans and Anglo American back-pain participants, the ANOVAs show that there were no statistically significant relationships between pain *intensity* variation and types of current pain medications, religion, gender, or SES. The best predictors of pain intensity variation in the combined study population were cultural-group identity, pain duration, and age. The native Puerto Rican group's intensity mean on the MPQ-PRIT was 47; the Anglo American group's mean of 31 was significantly lower (table 7.5). This difference between the two cultural groups remained in regression analysis when the influence of other variables, including age and duration, were controlled (see appendix F, table F.7, for the Regression table). The regression shows that as age rises, pain intensity goes down, and that as duration increases so does intensity. The R-square for this multiple regression equation was .416; thus, 42% of the variation in pain intensity in the combined population was explained by cultural identity, age, and pain duration.

Table 7.4. Significant Differences in Characteristics of Puerto Rican
and Anglo American Back-Pain Groups

Characteristic	Anglo American Group	Puerto Rican Group	F-ratio or Chi-Square
Religion (% of group)			11.90*
Catholic	45%	89%	
Protestant	55%	11%	
Age			43.85*
Mean	41.2	60.5	
Standard Deviation	14.3	11.2	
Pain Duration (in months)			48.86*
Mean	61.4	227.3	
Standard Deviation	83.9	121.9	

*$p < .01$

Inter-Cultural-Group Variation in Pain Responses

In addition to cultural differences in reported pain intensity, ANOVAs showed there were statistically significant inter-cultural-group differences in behavioral, psychological, and emotional responses to, and attitudes toward, chronic pain. (Multiple regressions also were performed on response areas that showed significant variations; included in each equation were the independent variables that were significantly related to inter- and intragroup differences in responses in the ANOVAs. In each response area discussed here, cultural background remained significantly associated with response differences in the regressions when the effects of other variables were controlled. For those readers interested in reviewing these regressions, they are located in appendix F, table F.8).

In the ANOVAs, there were no significant inter-cultural-group differences in any of the individual *daily activity* categories of sleeping, sex, walking, social activities, job, house chores, sports, and driving. Nor were there any in total interference with all daily activities (representing the total of all scores on the individual categories). There were also no significant differences between the two groups in degree of having to stop normal work inside and outside the home due to pain (work stoppage) (table 7.6).

There was a significant difference between the two cultural groups in the *behavioral response* area of expressiveness of the pain. The native Puerto Rican group scored a significantly higher mean (14.7 out of a possible 16) for degree of expressiveness than did the Anglo American group (mean 10.8 [see table 7.5]).

Table 7.5. Statistically Significant Inter-Cultural-Group Variations in Pain
Intensity and Behavioral, Psychological, and Attitudinal Responses

Response Area	Back Pain Anglo Americans	Back Pain Puerto Ricans	F-Ratio
Intensity (MPQ-PRIT)			27.9**
Mean	30.6	46.6	
SD	13.7	12.9	
Expressiveness[a]			10.78**
Mean	10.8	14.8	
SD	4.5	4.2	
Depression[a]			5.46*
Mean	2.9	3.6	
SD	1.1	1.0	
Worry[a]			2.89*
Mean	6.5	7.5	
SD	2.8	3.1	
Tension[a]			8.8**
Mean	3.1	3.8	
SD	1.1	0.7	
Pain = Unhappiness[b]			6.78**
Mean	1.6	2.5	
SD	0.9	1.4	
	Anglo Americans	Puerto Ricans	Chi-square
Health Attitude[c]			8.77**
Healthy	61%	25%	
Unhealthy/Disabled	39%	75%	

SD = Standard Deviation
*$p < .05$
**$p < .01$
[a]Pain-related degree of worry, tension, etc.; higher score means greater degree.
[b]Does patient believe that as long as pain persists his or her life will be unhappy? Higher
  scores indicate agreement that life will remain unhappy.
[c]Patient asked to define self as healthy or unhealthy/disabled.
Note: Many response scores are an aggregated score from several questions so the highest
  possible score varies by item.

In *psychological and emotional response areas*, there were significant
inter-cultural-group differences in degree of depression, worry, and tension associated with pain. The native Puerto Ricans had a significantly
higher self-reported degree of depression associated with their pain
(mean 3.6 out of a possible 4); the Anglo Americans' mean was 2.9 (see
table 7.5).

There also was a significant intergroup difference in degree of worry
associated with pain: the native Puerto Ricans scored a mean of 7.5 (out of

Table 7.6. Comparison of Interference in Daily Activities between Island Puerto Rican Back-Pain Group and Anglo American Back-Pain Group

	Anglo Americans (N = 48)	Island Puerto Ricans (N = 48)	F-Ratio	P^a
Work Stoppage				
Mean	5.1	5.2	0.05	.82
SD	2.3	1.6		
Total Interference in all Daily Activities				
Mean	29.4	29.9	0.13	.72
SD	5.3	6.6		
Interference with Sports				
Mean	3.9	3.7	0.63	.43
SD	.4	.8		
Interference with Social Activities				
Mean	2.9	3.0	0.09	.76
SD	.9	1.0		
Interference with House Chores				
Mean	3.3	3.5	1.59	.21
SD	.9	.7		
Interference with Driving				
Mean	3.0	3.0	0.05	.82
SD	1.0	1.1		
Interference with Walking				
Mean	3.0	3.0	0.02	.89
SD	.8	1.0		
Interference with Sexual Relations				
Mean	2.8	3.0	0.82	.37
SD	1.0	1.2		

SD = Standard Deviation
[a]There were no statistically significant differences in any daily activity categories.

12) compared to 6.5 for the Anglo Americans (table 7.5). In addition, the native Puerto Rican group also had a significantly higher mean for pain-related tension (see table 7.5 for actual means).

When assessing *attitudinal response* toward pain and happiness, the native Puerto Ricans' mean of 2.5, which indicated some agreement with the statement that pain means unhappiness, was significantly higher than the Anglo American group's mean of 1.6, which indicated some disagreement. In regard to attitudes toward health status, in the Anglo American group only 39% defined themselves as "unhealthy/disabled," while 75% of native Puerto Ricans defined themselves as "unhealthy/disabled" (table 7.5).

Intra-cultural-group differences in pain responses within the native Puerto Rican and Anglo American groups were discussed in chapters 5 and 6.

Qualitative Differences in the Context of Health Care

In addition to the quantitative differences in the chronic pain experiences of Puerto Rican and Anglo American participants, qualitative data reveal several clear differences in the context of health care between the Puerto Rican medical center and the New England center. On the island, healthcare providers viewed expressing pain as appropriate; thus, expressive patients in Puerto Rico met with no discrimination or disapproval. As mentioned in chapter 5, expressive Latino patients in New England did encounter disapproval from providers.

Also, the doctor-patient relationship on the island was conducted in a more personal manner, with much more attention given to the patient's family and social relationships and feelings concerning her or his pain and disease. In an interview, the center's chief physician said the best care he can provide to most chronic-pain and chronic-disease patients is to spend significant amounts of time with them and to listen, in an understanding manner, as the patients express their concerns, fears, anger, and frustrations. He said he believes such time is well spent because it results in improving patients' abilities to cope with their conditions.

A third and related area of difference in context was in the dominant worldview towards the mind-body relationship in the pain and illness experience. Puerto Rican physicians and patients share a holistic view of the pain experience and of mind-and-body integration. Physicians and the majority of patients expressed an understanding that emotional, psychosocial, and biological variables all interact in the pain experience, and patients generally accepted suggestions for psychological consultations or treatments without displaying anger. Angel and Guarnaccia also have argued that in traditional Puerto Rican culture "there is less of a separation of the psychological and physical senses of self" (1989:1234). Several subjects reported the simultaneous use of spiritists (traditional healers)[1] with medical center staff appearing to support such dual use of traditional and biomedical health-care resources. Also, probably as a result of this belief in mind-body integration, in the island Puerto Rican population the doctor's inquiries about family relationships and the patients' feelings about the pain and disability are seen as evidence of caring and concern for patients. Such inquiries about psychosocial aspects of the pain experience were not seen as indications that the doctor viewed the pain as *exclusively* stemming from psychological factors.

As noted in chapter 5, regarding Anglo Americans at the New England center, the physician's inquiries into psychosocial matters *were* seen as evidence that the doctor thought the pain was due to psychological factors, and therefore, in the patient's view, "not real." This interpretation is understandable as, although increasingly there are some biomedical literature acknowledgments of mind-body interactions, the dominant worldview of American biomedicine, as well as that of the majority of physicians at the New England center, remains one of mind-body dualism. Despite the marketing of a multidisciplinary approach to chronic pain management, at the New England center there was a continued preference (perhaps unconscious) on the part of physicians for biological diagnoses and biological treatments. Aware of this preference and also sharing a mind-body dualism worldview, patients were angered by suggestions that *their* pain related to psychological factors, and therefore they often resisted suggestions for psychological counseling.

Summary of Anglo American and Native Puerto Rican Comparison

In this cross-cultural comparison of the pain experiences of Anglo Americans and native Puerto Ricans, the factors found to be associated with significant differences were most often cultural or psychosocial factors, or related to the cultural context of care and treatment. The findings suggest that people from different cultural groups not only have different standards and meanings for pain but also have different overall percep-

---

1. Koss-Chioino (1992) offers a discussion of Puerto Rican Spiritists ("Espiritistas") and Spiritism. She also describes a collaborative project involving Puerto Rican mental health professionals, medical doctors, public health workers, and spiritists (Koss 1980, 1987; Koss-Chioino 1992).

tions of pain intensity and of the pain experience. However, despite the higher means for pain intensity and for emotional responses such as depression, worry, fear, and unhappiness, native Puerto Ricans as a group were not less functional in any of their daily activities (work, household chores, etc.). These studies suggest that, from emotional and cognitive perspectives, the two groups experience a different chronic pain reality which should be evaluated from an *emic* (insider or participant) perspective. Intragroup analyses are especially useful and necessary because they provide insight into the standards, norms, and range of variation within specific cultural groups.

In the final chapter, an integrated picture of the environment of the chronic pain sufferer will be presented, and recommendations will be made for more effective treatment and rehabilitation of multiethnic populations.

CHAPTER 8

SUMMARY AND CONCLUSIONS

Chronic pain is an experience that is affected by multiple factors. The two studies presented here clearly demonstrate considerable diversity among chronic pain patients. In contrast to the picture presented by many researchers and authors in the chronic pain field (Aronoff 1985:472; Kotarba 1983; Sternbach 1974; Lyndsay and Wyckoff 1981; Fordyce 1976), the two studies discussed here found that significant numbers of chronic pain patients have been and continue to be successful in adapting and adjusting their behaviors and attitudes to facilitate continuing or resuming meaningful and happy lives. Good (1992) also recently provided life stories of several professional women who had adapted to their chronic pain. The stories of pain sufferers who successfully adapt provide insight regarding successful coping strategies, which should be useful in improving treatment of other chronic pain sufferers.

Several of the factors that allowed study participants to adapt, or inhibited them from successfully adapting, to the chronic pain included degree of heritage consistency, generation, migration status, cultural gender-role expectations, and cultural meanings and standards for, and attitudes toward, pain and illness. The cultural context of health care also affected adaptation. Other influencing factors were patients' social networks or lack thereof, age, socioeconomic circumstances, and locus of control (LOC) styles and the political and economic contexts in which compensation, rehabilitation, employment, and health care were sought.

Chronic pain is a complex and poorly understood condition that often frustrates both providers and patients. The human and economic costs of chronic pain are enormous. Because physicians recognize there are currently no treatments that are effective for all pain sufferers, many providers need to be open to new approaches. However, in the United States today, the Anglocultural bias and the fragmented structure of the current system of health care, disability compensation, and rehabilitation are major deterrents to effective treatment of multicultural or multiethnic chronic pain populations. Effective treatment of chronic pain requires a better understanding of, and attention to, the overall environment of the chronic pain sufferer.

THE BIOCULTURAL ENVIRONMENT
OF THE CHRONIC PAIN SUFFERER

The quantitative analyses of these two studies and studies by others (McNeil, Sinkora, and Levavitt 1986; Jensen and Karoly 1991; Stenger 1992; Turk 1993) found little association between variation in pain intensity levels or pain responses and patients' specific diagnoses or current types of pain medications. Nonetheless, chronic pain patients still must be thoroughly evaluated diagnostically, and biomedical treatments that may provide pain relief and symptom reduction should be undertaken. The qualitative data in New England and in Puerto Rico show numerous instances in which patients' attributed substantial, although temporary, reductions in pain intensity and increases in activity levels to specific biomedical procedures such as steroid injections, intravenous lidocaine, or trigger-point injections. For many patients these respites of pain reduction and increased abilities to engage in activities were a great relief and allowed them to cope more effectively overall because they knew they could look forward to occasional periods when they felt better. (However, such treatments should be integrated with counseling and rehabilitation programs that address psychosocial and occupational aspects of the pain experience.)

For many patients in the two studies reported here, such as those with rheumatoid arthritis, even brief periods when pain and stiffness were lessened (as often occurred when steroids were injected directly into the affected joints) were very worthwhile. Many patients in Puerto Rico, including Maria in chapter 6, said they gained courage from the knowledge that when they went into severe "crisis" they could receive temporary relief by coming to the center for steroid injections. They understood such injections had to be spaced as far apart as possible due to long-term side effects, but the knowledge that temporary relief could be obtained at some point when the pain became unbearable helped them cope with their daily pain and disability.

In New England, those with arthritis and degenerative joint disease of the spine also reported temporary relief from steroid injections, and many patients with neuropathies or back pains reported similar temporary relief associated with their intravenous lidocaine treatments (see Jane's case in chapter 4). Thus, such biomedical treatments had more than an immediate effect: the knowledge of the temporary relief such treatments offered affected patients' attitudes. As with culturally related attitudes, these treatment-related attitudes may have a long-term effect on perceived pain intensity (through the supraspinal influences discussed in chapter 2), as well as on pain responses (such as degrees of depression, fear, and worry).

Therefore, the requirements for admission to many psychological/behavioral/cognitive pain treatment programs (especially the inpatient units) that patients must abandon the search for further biomedical diagnoses or treatments (Stans et al. 1989:318; Turk, Meichenbaum, and Genest 1983; Pither and Nicholas 1991) appear unwarranted and counterproductive. All aspects of the pain experience should be addressed in the treatment of chronic pain patients, and interactions among biological, psychosocial, cultural, and cognitive factors should be considered.

Obviously, different culturally prescribed styles of describing their pain may have affected the New England and Puerto Rican patients' reports of pain *severity* (chapters 4, 6 and 7). In the two studies, it was clear that members of the Anglo American and Polish groups tended to be less expressive or emotional when describing their pain than were members of the native Puerto Rican, New England Latino, and Italian groups. These differences appeared in both the qualitative and quantitative analyses. However, different reporting styles alone do not seem to explain the pain intensity differences or the correlations between intensity variation and degrees of depression and other psychological and attitudinal responses (see chapter 4, table 4.1).

As illustrated in the biocultural model (chapter 4, figure 4.4), in the complex process of human pain perception, socioculturally shaped attitudes, meanings, and degrees of attention may influence the neurophysiological processing of potentially pain-producing information as well as psychological, behavioral, and verbal responses to pain.

The biocultural model (figure 4.4) suggests that the source of social comparison is home and family, where adults transmit to children the values and attitudes of their cultural or ethnic group. Attitudes, expectations, meanings for experiences, and appropriate emotional expressiveness are learned through observing the reactions and behaviors of others who are similar in identity to oneself. The New England and Puerto Rican studies found significant ethnic or cultural differences in accepted standards for and attitudes toward pain and pain behaviors among defined ethnic groups.

In addition, Shorben and Borland (1954) found that children's dental phobias were directly influenced by the attitudes of their families toward dental care. Buss and Portnoy (1967), Craig and Neidermayer (1974),

Wooley and Epps (1975), and Linton and Gotestam (1985) also demonstrated that social modeling and group pressure influence pain tolerance levels. "There is also evidence that how a person defines his or her [pain] symptoms is largely based upon consultation with family members" (Turk, Flor, and Rudy 1987:3).

The biocultural model of pain perception does not assume any basic differences in the neurophysiology of members of different ethnic groups. People learn in social communities, where conventional ways of interpreting, expressing, and responding to pain are acquired. People with similar learning experiences are likely to show similar pain perception, expression, and response patterns. I term this patterning of pain perception and response as cultural. These culturally acquired patterns may influence the neurophysiological processing of nociceptive information as well a psychological, behavioral, and verbal responses to pain. These effects on the pain experience may occur through various supraspinal influences on pain perception discussed in detail in chapters 2 and 4.

Although it is likely that intense pain can affect attention, attitudes, and emotions, it is also possible that attitudes, degree of attention, and emotions were influencing perceptions of pain intensity in these two study populations. This is particularly plausible because, in the two studies reported here, pain intensity *variation* was not significantly associated with diagnosis, present medication types, or types of past treatments or surgeries for pain. Part of the variation in reported pain intensity among ethnic groups relates to different meanings, attitudes, beliefs, and emotional responses found in the different groups.

Therefore, if one is raised in a cultural environment which accepts and encourages (or on the other hand prohibits and discourages) an outward emotional expression of pain, or in one that defines focusing attention on the pain as either an appropriate or inappropriate response, these culturally acquired patterns not only may lead to certain styles of reporting, but also to different levels of perceived pain intensity.

The cross-cultural comparison of Anglo American and native Puerto Rican chronic pain sufferers suggest that people from different cultural environments not only have different standards and meanings for pain but also have different overall *perceptions of pain intensity* and of the pain experience. However, despite the higher means for pain intensity and on the psychometric measures for depression, worry, fear, etc., native Puerto Ricans as a group were not less functional in their daily social, work, and family lives than were the Anglo Americans. Qualitative and quantitative data reveal no significant differences between Anglo Americans and Puerto Ricans in interference in any of their work, social, or family activities (chapter 7, table 7.6).

In effect, as a group, Puerto Ricans simply appear to experience chronic pain differently from Anglo Americans—or, it could as easily be said that Anglo Americans appear to experience chronic pain differently from Puerto Ricans. The difference between groups is not positive or negative in itself—it is simply a different reality, which should be evaluated from an *emic* perspective and not through the cultural lens of the outside provider or researcher. Unfortunately, in clinical practice this is often not the case since the cultural reality of the provider guides her or his judgement of patients and treatment decisions. As a result, when pain sufferers are treated in a health-care environment dominated by a cultural group different from their own, the culturally shaped different realities of patients and providers lead to major communication problems and to significant stressors that adversely affect patients' abilities to adapt to their pain experiences.

However, within their own cultural environment, for native Puerto Rican patients and health-care providers alike, expressing, complaining, and focusing on pain is not inappropriate; rather, it is expected, normal, and acceptable. Furthermore, in keeping with their orientation toward reality, Latinos often accept that there are disagreeable aspects to life, such as illness, and they openly admit they do not like such experiences (Bastida 1979). So it is not surprising that the majority of Puerto Rican (and New England Latino) chronic pain participants openly defined their health status as unhealthy or disabled.

Despite this open acknowledgment of poor health; the open expression of pain; and associated tension, worry, and depression, many island Puerto Ricans involved in this study were functioning quite effectively and said they had good lives. Maria, whose case study was presented in chapter 6, is one clear example of this. She described how, during several "crisis" days, she not only cried out when in pain but got down on the floor and pounded her fists and screamed in anger and agony. Nonetheless, and overall, Maria clearly copes quite effectively with her arthritic pain and views herself as generally in control of both her pain and her life. Even with this positive attitude, though, Maria openly admits she wishes she did not have arthritis and describes her crisis days as very painful and exhausting.

In fact, when observational and coping strategies data on individuals' daily lives were assessed, many of those native Puerto Ricans, who psychometrically could be considered troubled, were actually highly productive.

If psychometric measures designed for Anglo populations or even those designed for cross-cultural use are interpreted by Anglo researchers or providers, the results may often lead to an interpretation that all

Latinos cope negatively with their pain experiences. However, Latinos' high scores on expressiveness, depression, worry, and tension are not necessarily indicators that they are coping poorly within their own cultural environment. When assessed by uninformed Anglo providers or researchers, however, these high psychometric scores may be misinterpreted due to a cultural bias that views expressing pain, complaining, and reporting one's worries and fears as negative outcomes rather than as acceptable expressions of a painful reality.

As the two studies show, cross-cultural comparisons are useful for documenting the role culture plays in the human pain experience. However, these two studies demonstrate that education and cultural sensitivity training of health-care providers must go beyond mere awareness. Indeed, a descriptive laundry-list approach to understanding cultural diversity, evident in some of the existing literature (for example Spector 1985), may only lead to stereotyping.

Therefore, *intragroup* analyses, which use both qualitative and quantitative methods, are an essential part of any cross-cultural or multiethnic study and also any effective clinical practice involving multiethnic populations. Intragroup analyses can be used to define the range of pain experiences, responses, and coping strategies within the specific cultural or ethnic group. Interpretations of scores on psychometric instruments and of interview materials can then be made within the framework of the specific ethnic or cultural group's range of variation.

A major component of the patient's assessment should be a detailed psychosocial and cultural history, taken by a provider or culture broker who is aware of both the complexity of biocultural and psychosocial variables in the chronic pain experience and of his or her own cultural background and biases. The work of Kleinman (1980, 1986, 1988) and Kleinman, Eisenberg, and Good (1978), regarding explanatory models and how to use a structured but open-ended interview to determine the meanings and explanations the patient attaches to the situation, would be helpful in effective history-taking and interpretation.

Such programs need to treat patients as individuals with specific biological, cultural, and psychosocial characteristics and cognitive interpretations that are likely to influence the chronic pain experience. Interpreters must be provided on a regular basis for patients who are not fluent in English, and assessment instruments (i.e., psychological tests, pain intensity and response measures) must be available in the clients' languages and tested for validity within the ethnic groups involved. Medical anthropologists, medical sociologists, or other culture brokers could be useful as consultants during history taking and in developing more effective chronic pain programs for multiethnic populations.

Within multiethnic or multicultural health-care environments, providers need to be informed by an understanding of the interactions of biology and culture in human pain perception and by an understanding of cultural relativity. They also need to be able to interpret results of patients' interviews and scores from psychometric instruments using the norms, patterns, and range of variation within the particular ethnic or cultural group rather than using standards of the provider's cultural group or of the culture of American biomedicine or Western psychiatry.

It should be stressed that culture does not affect patients alone. Medical providers' and specialists' own cultural backgrounds affect not only the communications and interactions between pain sufferer and health-care provider, but also the care and treatment provided. At the New England pain center, there were instances in which several nurses were judgmental toward the expressive Latinos and Italians; the nurses did not believe the expressiveness was appropriate—a judgment clearly related to the nurses' own cultural backgrounds. In addition, New England pain center physicians' preference for biological treatments was clearly related to the traditional worldview of the culture of biomedicine.

A study by Westbrook, Nordholm, and McGee (1984) compared evaluations of the same set of clinical patients' case histories by Swedish and Australian health-care providers. (These were not chronic pain patients.) The study found significant differences between the Swedish and Australian providers' evaluations and the treatment regimes they proposed. The authors attributed the dissimilarities to the different cultural backgrounds of the two sets of providers and the different health-care models of the medical education systems in Sweden and Australia. The study raises interesting questions about how providers' cultural and educational backgrounds influence their evaluation of patients and, subsequently, the care and treatment provided.

Like Westbrook, Nordholm, and McGee's, my studies suggest a need to investigate how providers' cultural and educational backgrounds affect the way they perceive, communicate with, care for, and treat chronic pain patients. Given the obvious stereotyping of such patients in much of the current literature, one can readily imagine how educational training that defines chronic pain patients as a homogeneous group with significant "psycho-socioeconomic disorders" (Aronoff 1985:472) would influence providers' perceptions and treatment of pain sufferers.

In biomedically oriented approaches to treating chronic pain, which were predominant at the New England pain center, there also has often been a continued reliance on the mind-body dualism bias. Inherent in the traditional culture of biomedicine, this bias creates contradictions between what chronic pain providers say and what they do. At the New

England pain center, physicians, nurses, and other providers verbally expressed a belief and commitment to a multidisciplinary, multicausal approach to understanding and treating chronic pain. However, in many (probably unconscious) ways their actions conveyed a continued belief in mind-body dualism, which often led to problems for patients (discussed in chapter 5). Fairly frequently, New England pain center staff gave contradictory messages about the relationship of mind and body in the chronic pain experience, which confused patients and inhibited their acceptance of psychosocial interventions.

At the New England pain center, despite the literature the center sent to each new patient concerning the center's multidisciplinary approach to understanding and treating chronic pain, which recognized the interaction of mind and body, when patients attended the center they observed a clear preference on the part of physicians for using biomedical procedures such as nerve blocks, epidural steroid injections, or intravenous medications. Often only after such procedures failed to bring pain relief did the New England physicians suggest to the patient that she or he should begin seeing the pain center psychologist for treatment. This suggestion was then interpreted by the patient as meaning the doctors no longer believed the pain was "real" (i.e., physical). (See Joe's case study in chapter 5 for such an example.)

Often long-term improvements in, for example, the Latino male patients' biopsychosocial condition might have been brought about if physicians and other staff had engaged in counseling patients about lifestyle and workplace changes while helping patients coordinate long-range strategies for job retraining or other forms of rehabilitation. Instead, physicians attempted to attain the immediate, and certainly not unworthy, goal of pain relief using biological approaches, which inevitably resulted in, at best, short-term improvements. Often within a week to a few weeks the severe pain returned and the biomedical procedure had to be repeated. Fordyce, Roberts, and Sternbach (1985) and Tollison et al. (1989) also have noted the tendency of traditional pain clinics to merely "treat the experience of pain and not the disability of pain" (Tollison et al. 1989:1125).

In contrast, as noted earlier, at the Puerto Rican center, physicians and patients viewed the mind and body as integrated in the pain experience. The Puerto Rican study confirmed a finding by Angel and Guarnaccia that in Puerto Rican culture "there is less of a separation of the psychological and physical senses of self" than in Anglo culture (1989:1234).

Furthermore, there is a strong Anglo cultural bias, as well as an element of social control, evident in the behavioral and cognitive approaches to chronic pain management. In these approaches the focus is not on reducing perceived pain intensity *per se* but on resocialization of the patient. In these approaches it is considered the patient's responsibility to suppress behavioral and verbal expressions of pain intensity or, in the cognitive approach, to redefine the pain as some other sensation or focus attention on other things and ignore the sensation of pain through the process of distraction. The goals of the relearning or resocialization process are to eliminate "deviant behaviors" such as not working and not meeting social obligations. One major goal is often to get the patients back to work (eliminating them from the disability rolls and counting them again as "productive" workers). Along with reinforcing the social value of work, the behavioral and cognitive approaches mirror Anglo American middle-class values related to the importance of "working" on a problem, taking individual responsibility for one's actions and problems, and remaining stoic and nonexpressive in the face of pain and adversity.

Such approaches not only ignore differences in beliefs and values among patients of varied ethnic and cultural backgrounds, but also place tremendous pressure on individual patients, who are told that only by changing their own actions and attitudes can the chronic pain be effectively treated (Holzman and Turk 1986). Although patients often still experience pain (Spence 1991), its source is no longer the focus of treatment. And, if unsuccessful at repressing or changing their pain behaviors and attitudes, or at replacing their "negative" cognitive perceptions of the pain with more "positive" interpretations, patients feel guilt and a sense of personal failure.

Another related cultural bias clearly evident in current treatment approaches to chronic pain is the adamant prescription that these patients must assume responsibility for their own pain and for changing pain behaviors. One has to question why chronic pain patients are singled out as being responsible for their own condition and own improvement. Acute pain patients, seen very differently in American biomedicine, are generally not held responsible for the existence and elimination of their pain. Yet because biomedicine has no clear way to alleviate chronic pain, it becomes the patients' responsibility. (Of course chronic pain is not the only ailment that is judged in this way; we see a similar judgmental approach to many AIDS patients and some cancer patients.)

This individualist, self-responsibility focus of many current types of chronic pain treatment programs is probably a product of the Anglo American cultural value on individual autonomy and belief that individuals have the potential, through their own efforts, to be anything they want to be (Bellah 1985; Finkler 1991; Rifkin 1987; Stein 1990; Tropman 1989; Wuthnow 1994). As noted in chapter 6, Marin and Triandis (1985:98) have identified the Anglo focus on the individual and individual goal attainment as an important element of cultural difference between Anglos and Hispanics/Latin Americans. They note that in contrast to the Anglo focus on the individual, Latin Americans and Hispanics place more stress on the collectivity and the necessity for collective action in goal attainment.

The Anglo belief (incorporated into modern biomedicine) in individual autonomy and the belief that through their own efforts alone individuals can attain any goals ignore the reality of life in a stratified, capitalist society such as the United States. Despite popular Anglo beliefs, economic and political forces and structural inequalities in such societies, as well as other social and physical environmental variables, have a tremendous impact on individuals' opportunities, circumstances, and health statuses. As Finkler (1991) notes:

> This [biomedical] model conceives of the person as an autonomous unit, independent of and isolated from other individuals and the social and cultural contexts. By not incorporating information about the family and the life world in which the patient is embedded, the medical consultation aggravates rather than allays the crisis for the patient. (126)

In the case of chronic pain, even inpatient chronic pain programs, which usually involve counseling of family members as well as patients, are insufficient because so many of the forces which affect the pain sufferer's experience are external to the patient and her or his family. In addition, occupational therapy's use of mechanical devices mirrors the mechanistic focus of the American biomedical model. In this respect, occupational therapy's treatments are similar to what is found in other areas of biomedicine, which generally focus on expensive mechanistic treatments of already existing diseases rather than on prevention or work and lifestyle changes that enhance health status (Waitzkin 1983:89–110; Bates 1990:252–256).

To effectively address these factors an ecological approach is needed that assesses and attempts to modify sociocultural, occupational, economic, and health-care elements of the overall environment (or "life world," as Finkler calls it) in which the pain sufferer lives, functions, and often must be employed.

It is true that such assessment and treatment will be expensive; however, in the United States, we are already spending vast sums of money on the care and treatment of chronic pain sufferers, yielding, at best, mixed to poor long-term results. The studies I have described demonstrate that culture is one of the major factors affecting the way people perceive and respond to chronic pain in themselves and in others. As long as the cultural backgrounds of both patients *and* providers are ignored in assessment and treatment programs, expensive treatments will remain ineffective for many. Long-term investment in educating health-care providers in personal cultural self-awareness, in self-awareness of the culture of biomedicine, and in cultural relativity may lead to more effective care and treatment and ultimately save money and reduce human suffering.

THE PSYCHOSOCIAL ENVIRONMENT OF THE CHRONIC PAIN SUFFERER

In the two studies described here, the most predominant psychological/cognitive factor affecting variation in the pain experience was locus of control (LOC) style. Others also have found significant relationships between subjects' LOC styles or views regarding control over life circumstances and variation in responses to pain, illness, or other stressful life events (Coreil and Marshall 1982; Afflek et al. 1987; Lefcourt 1980).

Furthermore, in these two studies LOC style was related to cultural background, as there was a significant difference in the distribution of the two LOC styles among the various ethnic and cultural groups (see chapter 3, figure 3.4). Except for the Anglo American group, ethnic identity was a predictor of LOC style. As it is impossible for LOC style to influence ethnic identity, probably socialization and psychosocial experiences as a member of a specific ethnic or cultural group has an effect on the LOC style one is most likely to develop. The two Latino groups in these studies had higher percentages in the external style than in any of the five non-Latino groups. As discussed in chapter 3, according to Ghali, the history of Puerto Rico's colonization and its current nebulous political status have left many island and mainland Puerto Ricans with a sense of powerlessness (1982:98). These historical and current political, social, and economic conditions combined with the Latin American cultural orientation toward reality may help explain why island Puerto Ricans and New England Latinos more often fall into the external LOC style than do members of non-Latino groups.

In these two studies there were statistically significant relationships between pain sufferers' LOC styles and variation in reported chronic pain intensity and responses (even when ethnic identity was statistically controlled). Such associations were also clear at the qualitative level, as among the themes that emerged in the qualitative data analyses was one involving patients' expressions of either having or lacking control over their pain and their current situations. This was a very common theme, which many patients mentioned in terms such as "I have no control over my life anymore," or "Once I got back control I felt better." This theme clearly relates to the LOC concept.

Qualitative data analyses revealed a pattern: the majority of patients reported that the first six to twenty-four months of the chronic pain experience involved severe changes in lifestyle and often involved a sense of having lost control of their lives. However, after this initial period, many patients seemed to diverge into two groups.

The first group was composed of patients who reported gradually regaining a sense of control and gradually adjusting successfully to the pain. This adjustment involved successful coping strategies, including restructuring or relocating their workplace or work schedules so they could return to former jobs or, when that was impossible, retraining for a new occupation, focusing on a new hobby, or "getting off" pain medications and using alternatives such as relaxation techniques (Bates and Rankin-Hill 1994; Bates, Edwards, and Anderson 1993; Bates et al. 1994). These successful coping strategies allowed patients in this group to adapt to pain and chronic disease, to once again find some purpose and pleasure in life, to stop the search for unrealistic cures, and to accept whatever degree of pain and disability could not be altered. The case studies of Manuel in chapter 1, Jane in chapter 4, Carl in chapter 5, and Maria in chapter 6 all demonstrate the various strategies used by those who exhibit a sense of control over their life circumstances.

Unlike these patients, the second group in the studies was composed of those who felt a lack of control over their lives. This group employed coping strategies—such as prescription drug dependency and a constant quest for a cure—but the results were generally unsatisfactory to patients, who remained in states of depression, anger, or frustration. Jesus, discussed in chapter 1; James and Mary, discussed in chapter 5; and Carlos in chapter 6 provide good examples of the pain experiences of those who lacked a sense of control over their lives.

When examining the qualitative data in association with the quantitative LOC scores, it was found that patients with an internal style were more likely to report that, after the initial period, they began to employ strategies which allowed regaining a sense of control, pleasure, and purpose in life. Those with an external style were more likely to be members of the group that employed strategies such as drug dependency or a continued unsuccessful search for an outside source (surgery, provider, or treatment) to "cure" them (Bates and Rankin-Hill 1994).

Qualitative data from these two studies also suggest that patients' LOC styles may change during the course of their chronic pain experiences; however, this suggestion is based solely on patients' retrospective reports of their sense of control prior to the pain experience. No pre-pain

LOC scores are available on any of the patients, and so their recollections of their sense of control prior to the chronic pain must be relied on. Therefore, a cause-and-effect relationship cannot be clearly established in respect to the correlation (i.e., statistically significant relationship) between LOC style and pain intensity variation, since the pain intensity, or the inability to control one's own pain intensity, may affect LOC style permanently or at various stages in the pain episode. On the other hand, LOC style may involve certain attitudes that influence pain perception. It can reasonably be suggested that differing attitudes associated with the two LOC styles may be affecting reported pain intensity perceptions in the New England and Puerto Rican study populations. Conceivably, attitudes associated with the two LOC styles alter pain perception in the same way as attitudes associated with the different ethnic or cultural groups. Ultimately, it seems likely that both as children and as adults, the differing attitudes toward control associated with the internal and external LOC styles develop and may be altered because of learning and psychosocial experiences in differing cultural, social, and/or physical environments and circumstances.

Numerous patients who reported a strong sense of control over their lives prior to the pain said they had gone through the six- to twenty-four-month period after the pain first began during which they felt a loss of control over their lives—a loss that grew out of their pain experiences. Patients who regained a sense of control after that initial period were able to "get on with life." Further intensive qualitative research is needed to document exactly what enabled such patients to regain a sense of control. However, thus far the interviews and case studies suggest that LOC style is not a permanent, unchanging characteristic and that therapeutic and rehabilitation programs can and should be developed to assist chronic pain patients to gain or reestablish a sense of control over their lives and their pain.

In light of the strong possibility that LOC style may be related to patients' abilities to adapt to the chronic pain experience, treatment programs initially should assess the patient's LOC style and the effects of that style on the patient's pain experience. Then, if it appears that an internal sense of control would be beneficial, providers should help the patient devise a program that offers *culturally appropriate* and *personally relevant* ways to develop or increase a sense of control over her or his circumstances. For example, developing effective and personalized occupational rehabilitation programs that help Latino male patients retrain for new occupations or help them restructure or relocate their work environments would provide a means for these patients to regain a sense of "manhood," self-worth, and self-control.

Furthermore, although the New England pain center and Puerto Rico studies found no statistically significant relationships between SES and LOC style, further research is needed on possible relationships and inter-actions between SES and LOC style in pain response variations. The fact that most patients at both study sites were working- to lower-middle class may be one reason why these studies found no significant relationships between LOC style and SES. Given that sufficient economic and material resources would appear to allow more control over the directions of one's life, at least in certain areas, further study involving populations with greater socioeconomic diversity is needed.

Degree of social support was also important to subjects' abilities to adapt to the chronic pain experience in these two studies and in other studies of health status (House, Landis, and Umberson 1990; Jacobson 1987). Participants with substantial support of family and friends reported lower degrees of pain-related stress. Especially for those who have insufficient social support, and for others as well, patient-led chronic pain support groups should be beneficial. Pain patients who cope success-fully should be recruited to assist with these groups. Such copers have much to offer others in the way of experienced-based advice on practical strategies for successful adaptation. They provide role models that illus-trate that chronic pain sufferers can have happy and fulfilled lives. Because a sense of control appears beneficial, I suggest that pain-sufferer-led groups may prove more useful than groups led by professionals. In many urban areas of the United States, chronic pain support groups are now available—although none existed at the New England pain center at the time of the study. Such groups are especially needed in Puerto Rico, where none have been available.

In addition to LOC style and degree of social support, other specific social and economic factors affected adaptation to chronic pain. These include age and SES (including educational, employment, and material circumstances). In general, the older age group (61 years and up) reported less-severe negative responses to chronic pain than did the youngest (20–40) and middle (41–60) age groups. Many in the oldest age group appeared to have adapted to living with chronic pain. Some possible rea-sons for the age differences were discussed in chapter 5. Probably those who were older (and thus were retired) did not have the day-to-day worry that when the pain was bad they would be unable to meet employ-ment or child-care obligations—thus, they may have experienced less stress than younger subjects who did have such obligations.

In regard to the influence of participants' SES on the pain experience, in these two studies subjects with higher levels of education and household income were more likely to still be working and expressed less worry and fear related to the pain experience than did subjects with lower levels of education and household income. Not surprisingly, sufficient economic resources and professional employment conditions appear to reduce pain-related work stoppage, fear, and stress.

THE EFFECTS OF THE POLITICAL AND ECONOMIC CONTEXTS OF HEALTH-CARE, COMPENSATION, AND REHABILITATION ON THE CHRONIC PAIN EXPERIENCE

In the New England pain center study population, 40% of the patients with chronic pain were receiving workers' compensation benefits and, therefore, their pain was attributed to on-the-job injuries. In Puerto Rico (where many subjects were retired), 25% of subjects were currently receiving workers' compensation benefits—so at least 25% of the subjects had chronic pain attributable to work-related injuries (the figure is probably higher, as some subjects who are now retired and not currently receiving workers' compensation were originally injured on the job). Clearly, conditions of employment that lead to worker injury are among the major causes of chronic pain in these two populations. More attention should be paid to prevention of chronic pain in workers through more rigorous workplace safety programs. Especially since there is no known cure for chronic pain, more focus on prevention of workplace injury would create savings in human suffering as well as in health-care costs and workers' compensation expenses.

Subjects who were receiving workers' compensation benefits were more likely to report higher degrees of work stoppage, both inside and outside the home, and higher degrees of overall interference in daily activities than were noncompensation subjects. Those receiving workers' compensation were more likely to have immediately sought the care of a medical doctor when the pain began and more likely to have reported following doctors orders than noncompensation patients. Within some ethnic groups, those receiving workers' compensation reported greater unhappiness and believed less that they could ultimately overcome the pain than those not receiving compensation.

The significant relationships between workers' compensation status and patients' behavioral and attitudinal responses were not surprising. Subjects receiving workers' compensation often reported substantial difficulties in obtaining their benefits and great fears that any physical activity on their part could lead to loss of benefits and thus to personal financial disaster. The vast majority of these patients had significant low-back problems or other serious medical diagnoses; they were not "malingerers."[1]

This fear of engaging in physical activities is very detrimental to chronic pain patients, as studies have shown that those sufferers who remain active often reported less-severe pain and disability (Wall and Jones 1991:213; Tollison et al. 1989; Osterweis, Kleinman, and Mechanic 1987:236). However, under adversarial circumstances, the fears patients expressed seemed appropriate responses to a system which, despite its original intent, currently often favors profitmaking over providing compensation and support to workers with job-related injuries. Under such a system then, it is not surprising that those receiving workers' compensation immediately sought a doctor's care to document their injuries, reported higher levels of interference in daily activities and higher levels of unhappiness, and were more likely to express fears that they might not overcome their pain.

Those on private disability benefits did not necessarily fare any better than workers' compensation recipients. Jesus's case, discussed in chapter 1, involved private disability benefits because his back problems were not related to an on-the-job injury. His employer offered professionals such as Jesus not only workers' compensation coverage but private disability insurance for non-job-related injuries or illness. Jesus experienced numerous problems with his disability insurer who, for instance, refused to cover costs for him to stay at a live-in chronic pain treatment and rehabilitation center on the mainland which the physician had recommended. (A study by Tollison et al. [1989] found that workers' compensation insurance companies often also denied recipients funding for evaluation and treatment at chronic pain treatment centers.) In Jesus's case, the disability insurer also was unable to gain the cooperation of his former employer when the physician and Jesus suggested a trial twenty-hour work week. Jesus was devastated by this refusal.

---

1. At both study sites, the vast majority of the patients had significant injuries or diseases that contributed to their chronic pain. I encountered very few patients who could be considered "malingerers." Despite the public perception that people on workers' compensation or other forms of disability often are trying to "milk the system," this research did not find a high rate of such people. For those below retirement age who had to cease employment due to the pain, the vast majority wanted to go back to work, and many of them desperately wanted to do so as they found life without employment to be boring and unfulfilling as well as financially difficult.

Patients' abilities to adapt to their chronic pain experiences also were affected by the political and economic context of the health-care setting. Political and economic conditions within the health-care institution affected care and treatment, as they determined what services were available at the institution. For example, at the New England pain center, despite recognition that translation services in Spanish would improve the care and treatment of Latino patients, the director was unable to initiate such services due to institutional budget constraints.

Counseling New England patients on lifestyle and workplace changes and providing advocacy services related to workers' compensation and rehabilitation services often would have been as beneficial as biomedical procedures, but they generally were not provided. It must be acknowledged that institutional constraints on providers made lengthy counseling of patients extremely difficult at the New England pain center. As previously noted, during the research period the administration of the medical center reduced the number of pain center physicians, as well as the number of nursing hours. At the same time, the New England pain center was supposed to continue to increase patient load. These policies increased the workplace stress on the health-care providers and obviously decreased the time that nurses and doctors could spend with individual patients. Under such circumstances it is understandable that providers failed to provide in-depth counseling to patients.

In addition, political and economic considerations shaped the delivery of occupational therapy services at both study sites. Many patients at both sites wanted to return to work, but often occupational therapy services did not actively help patients with this goal. At the New England pain center and in Puerto Rico, occupational therapy programs often prescribed and provided devices and appliances to increase ability to engage in tasks of daily living rather than offering long-range counseling and coordination of services for returning to work. Time spent counseling patients on retraining or coordinating their return to work may be less profitable for health-care institutions than prescription and sale of hardware. Health-care provision in the United States is, after all, a major for-profit industry—so the trend toward the use of expensive mechanistic approaches is not surprising. Furthermore, of course, the occupational therapy focus mirrors the mechanistic worldview of biomedicine.

While occupational therapy programs on the island appeared to be as ineffective as in New England at helping patients return to work, at the Puerto Rican medical center the chief physician did spend time counseling patients on social and economic matters and functioned also as a patient advocate. He often wrote appeals when patients' workers' compensation or Social Security Disability Insurance (SSDI) benefits were denied and in some cases wrote the disability insurer asking that the patient's former employer make accommodations for the person to return to work at least part-time.

Finally, at the New England pain center, despite the claims in the center's literature and by its staff that it operated as a multidisciplinary treatment facility, there often appeared to be insufficient coordination between the various programs offered. Individual physicians worked at the New England pain center one to two days a week (and in other departments the rest of the week), so patients could only see the same physician consistently if they were able to come on the same day of each week. As this was not always possible, many patients saw different physicians during repeat visits and had no single physician who oversaw their case on a regular basis or coordinated and evaluated their treatment through the various programs and services.

Weekly staff meetings, involving members of the various programs and services, were held in which specific patients' progress and treatments were evaluated and altered if deemed appropriate. (I occasionally attended and observed these meetings, recording fieldnotes after each occasion.) Time often ran out before all of the week's cases could be discussed, and there was no established schedule for reevaluating each current patient on a regular basis. As a result, with the exception of "problem patients" whose cases often were addressed at the weekly meetings because of providers' frustrations, fairly frequently patients had no physician or staff member who periodically evaluated the effectiveness of various treatments.

Furthermore, on numerous occasions, I observed patients attempting to gain physicians' assistance with workers' compensation or other disability claims and, more often than not, physicians made it clear they did not like to have to deal with such matters and did not appreciate the gatekeeping function assigned to them under the current compensation and disability systems. Often patients left papers to be filled out by attending physicians, only to have them never returned to the insurers. When repeated appeals by phone or during regularly scheduled visits failed to bring about results, some patients would sit for hours in the waiting room trying to get an opportunity to see a doctor personally to obtain compensation-related evaluations. Thus, coordination of internal services as well as coordination and cooperation with other agencies the pain sufferer relied on for financial and rehabilitative assistance were sometimes insufficient at the New England pain center.

At both the quantitative and qualitative levels these two studies found that conditions of present or former employment and of subjects' workers' compensation or other disability status affected pain sufferers' responses to their situation and their abilities to successfully adapt to their situations. In the current U.S. system of employment, compensation, rehabilitation, and health care, there is a severe lack of coordination and cooperation among various agencies and services that is detrimental to many chronic pain sufferers (and others with disabilities).

The United States has several different disability programs, which "were created in isolation from one another and continue to run separately" (Berkowitz and Berkowitz 1989:209). SSDI is a nearly invisible part of the Social Security Program, paid for by Social Security contributions of both workers and employers. SSDI is "designed to provide [disability] benefits to those who have been employed but are no longer able to work because of medically determined impairment" (Osterweis, Kleinman, and Mechanic 1987:37).

SSDI is not for on-the-job injuries but for people who have worked under Social Security and become disabled through disease or non-job-related injuries. Former workers are not eligible for SSDI benefits unless they have an impairment that prevents them "from engaging not only in [their] previous work but in any kind of work that exists in the national economy, taking into account the claimant's age, education and work experience" for at least twelve consecutive months (Osterweis, Kleinman, and Mechanic 1987:39). For many applicants the process of obtaining SSDI benefits is lengthy and often involves initial denial and repeated appeals.

The vocational rehabilitation program of the federal government is a relatively obscure program with a modest ($1 billion) annual budget, paid for through general revenues (Berkowitz and Berkowitz 1989:210). The aim of this program is job retraining, and those who receive SSDI benefits are required by provisions to seek services of the vocational rehabilitation program. However, as Osterweis, Kleinman, and Mechanic (1987) note,

> there appears to be a serious "catch-22"—to be eligible for [SSDI] disability benefits a claimant must prove that he or she is unable to engage in any substantial gainful employment that exists in the national economy because of medical impairment that is expected to either last for at least 12 months or to end in death. To be eligible for rehabilitation a claimant must demonstrate both the potential for work and that rehabilitation would be beneficial. In light of these conflicting requirements, it does not seem surprising that the rehabilitation provisions are rarely used and that few people ever go off the [SSDI] disability rolls by returning to work. (70)

A further impediment to rehabilitation is the often lengthy delay of the appeals process for SSDI. By the time SSDI benefits are finally obtained, several years may have passed since the original injury or illness began, even though repeated studies show that rehabilitation services are most effective when received in the early stages of the disability (Osterweis, Kleinman, and Mechanic 1987; Berkowitz and Berkowitz 1989; Talo, Hendler, and Brodie 1989).

I encountered only a few patients at the New England pain center who had access to the state's rehabilitation services. Those who did were usually receiving SSDI benefits rather than workers' compensation and tended to have had chronic pain for extended periods before gaining access to rehabilitation services. The case of James, presented in chapter 5, is one example. By the time they gained access to rehabilitation services, the chronic pain and associated disability were of long duration and appeared resistant to long term improvements; thus, patients such as James were caught in the "Catch-22" described by Osterweis, Kleinman, and Mechanic.

Some employers also offer private disability insurance to employees, or individuals may purchase such insurance from a variety of insurers—many of whom are for-profit U.S. insurance companies. This private insurance covers disability from illness or non-job-related injuries and typically offers replacement of workers' salary up to approximately 60% of former income; many also offer medical benefits. These private policies often have very strict definitions of disability and require claimants to also apply for SSDI benefits; "some will not provide benefits to people who are not receiving public benefits" and the private benefits are generally reduced by the amount of the public benefits paid the individual (Berkowitz and Berkowitz 1989:213–214). The individual is usually subject to lengthy appeals before both public and private disability insurers before they receive the private insurance wage-replacement benefits. Private insurers often may also deny expensive health-care benefits.

If a worker's "illness or injury occurs in the course of employment, a completely different program, workers' compensation, applies" (Berkowitz and Berkowitz 1989:210). This state-level, rather than federal-level, program, paid for through employers' contributions, covers medical costs for temporary or permanent or partial or complete disabilities, as well as some costs of rehabilitation services, and provides loss-of-salary damages. By law, state workers' compensation programs must be provided and were originally developed, at least in theory, "to protect employees, spare them from the uncertainties of the judicial system and limit the legal liability of employers" (211). Most states allow employers to "buy their workers' compensation insurance from private [for-profit] carriers, or simply to self-insure" (211). Despite the original intent to spare workers from the "uncertainties of the judicial system," my research suggests that there are often lengthy hearings before state workers' compensation boards before workers are granted benefits and, if appeals to the state boards fail, workers may still have to pursue their claims in court.

In the two studies described in this book, one of the major factors affecting many pain sufferers has been the adversarial relationship created by the often lengthy process of obtaining workers' compensation, SSDI, or private disability benefits, or pursuing other forms of litigation. This process has inhibited patients' from engaging in physical activities they might have been capable of doing and from participating in early rehabilitation.

Others have reported similar patterns (Tait, Chibnall, and Richardson 1990; Talo, Hendler, and Brodie 1989; Osterweis, Kleinman, and Mechanic 1987). Talo, Hendler, and Brodie's study found that some workers' compensation patients fear "going out of the house. . . . [The] fear that their real disabilities will not be taken seriously hinders them in too 'visible' activities." They conclude: "it may be that the system is creating its own vicious circle" (1989:269). Tait, Chibnall, and Richardson (1990) also mention the "adversarial nature of the Workers' Compensation system" (37), and Osterweis, Kleinman, and Mechanic (1987) discuss the detrimental effects of this adversarial relationship between disability programs and applicants on the rehabilitation process.

As Osterweis, Kleinman, and Mechanic note, the current SSDI system and many private disability insurance plans take an all-or-nothing approach to disability. One is totally and permanently disabled and incapable of reentry into the labor force and, therefore, eligible for disability benefits and, paradoxically, rehabilitation benefits; or, one is defined as not disabled, capable of some type of work (even if it is not the work they originally did), and thus not entitled to such benefits. This system is not flexible and innovative enough to provide the disabled with trial attempts at integration back into the workforce—at least not without threatening permanent loss of benefits if the trial fails. This is especially unfortunate; several of the case studies in this book illustrate that people with fairly severe disabilities and chronic pain can function effectively in the world of employment if appropriate physical modifications in the work setting are made and if work schedules provide flexibility.

An additional factor affecting chronic pain patients is often not openly discussed in the existing medical literature. This factor is the profit motive. The desire for profits on the part of compensation and disability insurers, former employers, and health-care providers and facilities affects how chronic pain patients are treated and what they receive for rehabilitation opportunities and treatments.

While many European countries incorporate the workers' compensation benefit system into their governments' overall social security systems or national health-insurance systems (Roemer 1991)—thereby *not* tying workers' compensation benefits to a for-profit insurance industry—in the United States, workers' compensation insurance is not part of the government Social Security system. Rather, workers' compensation insurance is often provided through for-profit insurance companies. The main goal of these companies is profit, and thus the companies seek to deny claims or keep health-care and wage-replacement payments as low as possible while still maintaining insurance accounts.

Much of the private disability insurance in the United States is also sold through for-profit insurance companies. For these insurers, short-term profits are often more important than long-term savings. Thus, claimants such as Jesus are often denied funds for treatment at inpatient rehabilitation centers, even though studies have demonstrated that, for some, inpatient programs that offer comprehensive treatment result in long-term savings on future health care and often lead to a return to work (Tollison et al. 1989:1116). As mentioned above, the two studies described in this book show that even if the insurer pays for pain control center treatment, there often is a lack of coordination and cooperation among the pain center's programs, the compensation insurer, and the former employer.

In addition, former employers are often unwilling to provide workplace changes or flexible work schedules; again, the profit motive is probably involved. For example, in Puerto Rico, when his physician wrote the appeal for schedule flexibility so that Jesus could return to part-time work, Jesus's former employer was unwilling to cooperate. The current high rate of unemployment on the island (and on the mainland as well) contributes to employers' inflexibility, since, given the ample supply of workers—including white collar professionals—it often may seem simpler and cheaper to hire a new person than to make accommodations for a disabled worker. In Jesus's case, the employer probably believed it was less costly to replace him (he had over twenty years with the company and was earning a high salary when he left) with a less experienced lower-paid employee.

CONCLUSIONS AND RECOMMENDATIONS

In conclusion, clearly the overall biocultural, psychosocial, political, economic, and health-care environment of the chronic pain sufferer must be assessed and, in many cases, altered if the patient is to adjust successfully and adapt to the chronic pain and associated disease or disability. Yet the present fragmented, poorly coordinated, profit-oriented U.S. system of health-care, psychological counseling, compensation, and rehabilitation makes it very difficult to address the multiple needs of chronic pain populations.

Culturally appropriate health-care and psychological services must be coordinated with more effective long-term strategies for rehabilitation. The cooperation of former employers is also essential in cases where the patient has the potential for returning to some type of meaningful work—at least part-time. If the patient was not formerly employed, is permanently retired, or is disabled to the extent that no employment is possible, rehabilitation services are still essential as such patients often need assistance in altering the home and social environments to facilitate participation in activities that are meaningful and important to them.

The coordination of services will be a complex process and will require the services and close cooperation of a primary care physician or case manager for each patient. (Upon discharge, inpatient chronic pain services often provide some follow-up visits and/or evaluations; however, long-range case management of discharged patients is not typical.) As there currently is an under-supply of general practitioners in the United States, the patient often has no primary-care physician to coordinate services, put the entire picture together, and assist the patient in obtaining services and cooperation from the multiple agencies and institutions involved. Yet, the two studies described in this book and others suggest that continuity of care is beneficial to chronic pain patients (Sheridan 1992:146).

I suggest that a case-manager approach would be a cost-effective way of providing coordination of services while at the same time providing the pain sufferer with a supportive long-term relationship with a skilled advocate. (Because of providers' frustrations when dealing with chronic pain, many of these pain patients have experienced significant distress from unsatisfactory relationships with providers, so the importance of a sensitive, knowledgeable, and supportive advocate cannot be overstressed.)

Because this research indicates that a sense of control is beneficial to the process of positive adaptation to chronic pain and disease in patients from varied cultural backgrounds, patients should be encouraged to play an active role in this process, gaining a sense of control over the direction of their treatment and rehabilitation. Thus, the relationship between the case manager (who should be trained in cultural relativity and cultural self-awareness) and patient should be that of partners working together to create the best possible solution for the particular patient—a solution which leads the patient to a life he or she defines as meaningful and worthwhile. The case manager should, however, provide emotional support as well as professional services as these and other studies show the beneficial effects of social support on health.

Since the process of adaptation to chronic pain and disease requires continual adjustments as circumstances in the internal and external environments change, the case-manager/patient relationship should be an ongoing one in which both periodically assess, discuss, and plan appropriate strategies as needed. Chronic pain patients who are coping successfully should not be excluded from case-management services, since adaptation is an ongoing process. Counseling and supporting such patients can help them adjust to changes as they occur and assist them in coping with inevitable crises in order to prevent long-term problems. Although a culturally sensitive, ecologically focused, case-manager approach to the treatment and rehabilitation of chronic pain sufferers initially will be expensive, such a strategy will result in long-term savings in human suffering, health-care expenses, and disability benefits.[2]

The case-manager approach and greater use of self-help chronic pain support groups are suggested as microlevel strategies. At the macrolevel, in the years ahead as the United States restructures its health-care system and mechanisms for financing health insurance, attention should be given to designing an overall system which integrates workers' compensation and other disability programs with effective rehabilitation and health care. For long-term improvements, the current fragmented U.S. system, with its many contradictions and deincentives for rehabilitation, must be replaced by an integrated system that establishes cooperation between services and provides a supportive context in which patients can pursue rehabilitation or retraining without fearing financial disaster from losing necessary compensation and health benefits. Such a system should also take a preventive approach to workplace injury.

----

2. Tollison et al. (1989) report on an industrial-medicine approach to inpatient chronic pain treatment that appears to address many of these multiple needs; however, the program completely fails to consider cultural or ethnic background of patients or providers.

APPENDIX A
ETHNICITY AND PAIN SURVEY
Dr. Maryann S. Bates Copyright 1988

1. What religious tradition would you say most closely typifies your childhood?

_____ Protestant
_____ Catholic
_____ Jewish
_____ Agnostic/atheist
_____ Other, please specify _____

2. Were *you*, either of *your parents*, or *any of your grandparents* born in a country other than the United States, and if so where? no _____ yes _____

Who (e.g., mother, father, maternal grandmother, etc.)?
Where born?

_____

_____

_____

_____

3. Do you consider yourself to be a member of any of these ethnic groups? (Please check the one group you see as your primary affiliation and any other you consider to be secondary.)

	Primary	Secondary
Irish	_____	_____
African-American	_____	_____
Hispanic	_____	_____
Polish	_____	_____
French Canadian	_____	_____
Italian	_____	_____
Other Group	_____	_____
Please Specify	_____	

4. When you were growing up, what language was spoken in your home? Please Specify _____

5. What is your date of birth? _____
    month   day   year

159

APPENDIX B
McGILL PAIN QUESTIONNAIRE

Some of the words below describe your present pain. Circle ONLY those words that best describe it. Leave out any category that is not suitable. Use only a single word in each appropriate category – the one that applies best.

1.	Flickering	_____
	Quivering	_____
	Pulsing	_____
	Throbbing	_____
	Beating	
	Pounding	_____

2.	Jumping	_____
	Flashing	_____
	Shooting	

3.	Pricking	_____
	Boring	_____
	Drilling	_____
	Stabbing	_____
	Lancinating	_____

4.	Sharp	_____
	Cutting	_____
	Lacerating	_____

5.	Pinching	_____
	Pressing	_____
	Gnawing	
	Cramping	_____
	Crushing	_____

6.	Tugging	_____
	Pulling	_____
	Wrenching	_____

7.	Hot	
	Burning	_____
	Scalding	_____
	Searing	_____

8.	Tingling	_____
	Itchy	_____
	Smarting	
	Stinging	

9.	Dull	_____
	Sore	_____
	Hurting	_____
	Aching	_____
	Heavy	_____

10.	Tender	_____
	Taut	_____
	Rasping	_____
	Splitting	_____

| 11. | Tiring | _____ |
| | Exhausting | _____ |

| 12. | Sickening | _____ |
| | Suffocating | _____ |

13.	Fearful	_____
	Frightful	_____
	Terrifying	_____

161

14.	Punishing	_____	18.	Tight	_____
	Gruelling	_____		Numb	_____
	Cruel	_____		Drawing	_____
	Vicious	_____		Squeezing	_____
	Killing	_____		Tearing	_____

15. Wretched _____
    Blinding _____

16. Annoying _____
    Troublesome _____
    Miserable _____
    Intense _____
    Unbearable _____

17. Spreading _____
    Radiating _____
    Penetrating _____
    Piercing _____

19. Cool _____
    Cold _____
    Freezing _____

20. Nagging _____
    Nauseating _____
    Agonizing _____
    Dreadful _____
    Torturing _____

PPI
0 No Pain _____
1 Mild _____
2 Discomforting _____
3 Distressing _____
4 Horrible _____
5 Excruciating _____

PRI (T) $\overline{(1-20)}$

M(T) $\overline{(17-20)}$

M(AE) $\overline{(20)}$

M(S) $\overline{(17-19)}$

E $\overline{(16)}$

A $\overline{(11-15)}$

PRI: S $\overline{(1-10)}$

SPANISH McGILL PAIN QUESTIONNAIRE

Tab. 1: Adaptation to Spanish of MPQ verbal Descriptors.

SENSORIAL

1. Temporal
   1. Aleteo
   2. Palpitación
   3. Latido
   4. Golpeteo
   5. Martilleo

2. Espacial
   1. Sobresalto
   2. Fulgurante
   3. Latigazo

3. Presión Puntiforme
   1. Punzada
   2. Agujereo
   3. Taladranté
   4. Puñalada
   5. Lancinante

4. Presión Incisoria
   1. Agudo
   2. Cortante
   3. Lacerante

5. Presión Constrictiva
   1. Pellizco
   2. Opresión
   3. Roedor
   4. Calambre
   5. Estrujamiento

6. Presión por Tracción
   1. Tirón
   2. Sacudida
   3. Retorcimiento

7. Térmico
   1. Caliente
   2. Quemante
   3. Hirviente
   4. Abrasador

8. Brilio
   1. Hormilgueo
   2. Picor
   3. Resquemor
   4. Escozor

9. Matídez
   1. Sordo
   2. Dolorimiento
   3. Hiriente
   4. Profundo
   5. Duro

10. Sensorial: Miscelánea
    1. Sensible
    2. Tenso
    3. Aspero
    4. Terebrante

```
AFECTIVO                    EVALUATIVO

11. Tensión                 16.
    1. Fatigoso                 1. Molesto
    2. Agotador                 2. Fastidioso
                                3. Agoblante
                                4. Intenso
                                5. Insoportable
12. Autonómico
    1. Nauseante
    2. Asfixiante
                            MISCELÁNEA

                            17.
13. Miedo                       1. Se extiende
    1. Temible                  2. Se irradia
    2. Pavoroso                 3. Penetrante
    3. Aterrador                4. Traspasante

                            18.
                                1. Apretado
                                2. Entumecido
14. Castigo
    1. Mortificante
    2. Penoso               19.
    3. Despiadado               1. Frescor
    4. Maligno                  2. Frio
    5. Mortal                   3. Helado

                            20.
                                1. Pertinaz
15. Afectivo-Evaluativo-        2. Repugnante
    Sensorial: Miscelánea       3. Atroz
    1. Ingrato                  4. Espantoso
    2. Cegador                  5. Torturante
```

Tab. 2: Adaptation to Spanish of MPQ verbal intensity scale

```
1. Leve
2. Incómodo
3. Angustioso
4. Horrible
5. Aniqullador
```

APPENDIX C
ETHNICITY AND PAIN QUESTIONNAIRE
Dr. Maryann S. Bates   Copyright 1988

Section A:

(1) Where is your pain located? _____

(2) What is the cause of your pain? _____

(3) Do you think you have a clear explanation for your pain? _____

(4) How long have you had your pain? _____

(5) How long have you been coming to your physician for
    treatment? _____

Section B: For each question or statement below please indicate
         your answer by circling the number code beside the
         answer that comes closest to your response.

        0=not applicable
        1=disagree strongly
        2=disagree somewhat
        3=agree somewhat
        4=agree strongly

(6) I still have many of the same friends
     that I had as a child or teenager.   0 1 2 3 4

(7) I live in the same neighborhood as I
     did during my childhood (or I was born
     in my country of origin and later immi-
     grated to the U.S. mainland).   0 1 2 3 4

(8) Most of my friends live in the same
     neighborhood that I do.   0 1 2 3 4

(9) I see and socialize with my brothers,
     sisters, or parents on a regular basis. 0 1 2 3 4

(10) I still identify with the ethnic or
     cultural traditions of my childhood,
     and those traditions still play a role
     in my present lifestyle.   0 1 2 3 4

(11) I often tell others about my pain.   0 1 2 3 4

(12) It helps me if I talk about my pain.   0 1 2 3 4

(13) I become very emotional when I describe
     my pain to doctors and to other people. 0 1 2 3 4

0=not applicable
1=disagree strongly
2=disagree somewhat
3=agree somewhat
4=agree strongly

(14) When the pain gets bad I may moan
or groan.   0 1 2 3 4
(15) I cannot hide my pain from others.   0 1 2 3 4
(16) My pain has made it impossible for me
to carry on with the work I did before
I had it.   0 1 2 3 4
(17) As soon as the pain began I stopped
work and stayed at home.   0 1 2 3 4
(18) While I have had to revise my activity
schedule because of the pain, I have
been able to find new activities or
work that keep me busy and active.   0 1 2 3 4
(19) My pain makes me worry about what is
wrong with me.   0 1 2 3 4
(20) I think a lot about my pain.   0 1 2 3 4
(21) My major fear is that I may have cancer
or some other serious disease.   0 1 2 3 4
(22) I think a lot about what I could have
done to deserve my pain.   0 1 2 3 4
(23) Once the real reason for my pain is
discovered I will worry less, even if
I still have pain.   0 1 2 3 4
(24) When I am in pain I feel very tense.   0 1 2 3 4
(25) When I am in pain I feel very angry.   0 1 2 3 4
(26) I feel very afraid when I am in pain.   0 1 2 3 4
(27) I become depressed when I am in pain.   0 1 2 3 4
(28) I am determined that I will overcome
my pain.   0 1 2 3 4
(29) As long as I am in pain I will never
have a fulfilling and happy life.   0 1 2 3 4
(30) When I first had pain I went to a
medical doctor right away.   0 1 2 3 4
(31) I do not believe in taking medicine
for pain.   0 1 2 3 4
(32) If a doctor says medicine will help me,
then I take it exactly as directed.   0 1 2 3 4
(33) I have been to a chiropractor.   0 1 2 3 4
(34) If a doctor gives me medicine or tells
me to do something and it does not help
within a few days, I stop taking the
medicine or discontinue the treatment.   0 1 2 3 4

0=not applicable
1=disagree strongly
2=disagree somewhat
3=agree somewhat
4=agree strongly

(35) I have asked my friends and relatives
     how I should treat pain problems and
     have tried remedies they suggested.   0 1 2 3 4
(36) I have turned to friends or relatives for
     help while I have had my pain problem.   0 1 2 3 4
(37) My friends and relatives have been
     supportive during the times I have
     had problems with pain.   0 1 2 3 4

Section C.

(38) Do you consider yourself to be (a) healthy   _____
                                   (b) unhealthy _____
                                   (c) disabled   _____
                                   (d) other _____
                                              (please specify)

Section D. Please indicate whether or not you think each item
           below is true or false by circling T for true and F for
           false. (True is scored as 1 False is scored as 0.)

(39) People's misfortunes usually result from the
     mistakes they make.   T   F
(40) Unfortunately, an individual's worth often
     passes unrecognized no matter how hard he
     or she tries.   T   F
(41) Many of the unhappy things in people's lives
     are partly due to bad luck.   T   F
(42) Making a decision to take a definite course of
     action has usually worked better for me than
     trusting to fate.   T   F
(43) I have often found that what is going to
     happen will happen and that I do not have
     control over many things that happen to me.   T   F
(44) Succeeding at most things is a matter of hard
     work; luck has little or nothing to do with it.   T   F
(45) When I make plans, I am almost certain that I
     can make them work.   T   F
(46) Many times I feel that I have little influence
     over the things that happen to me.   T   F

(47) Much of the time I feel that I do not have
     enough control over the direction my life
     is taking.   T   F
(48) I believe that I control my pain rather
     than that my pain controls my life.   T   F

APPENDIX D

Estudio Investigativo Acerca de la Etnicadad y de Dolor

1. ¿Qué tradición religiosa mejor describe su religión de crianza?
   _____ Protestante
   _____ Católica
   _____ Judía
   _____ Agnóstica/Atea
   _____ Otra (Favor de especificar) _____

2. ¿Nació usted, o sus padres o abuelos, en algón país que no sea
   los Estados Unidos?   Sí _____ No _____

¿Quién (indique abuela o abuelo por parte de madre o de padre, etc.?
¿En qué país? _____
_____
_____

3. Indique en la primera columa con qué groupo se identifica usted
   principalmente. Si hay otra grupo con el cual usted también se
   identifica, indique su grupo secundario en la otra columa.

	Grupo Principal	Grupo(s) Secundario(s)
Puertorriqueño	_____	_____
Negro	_____	_____
Hispano	_____	_____
Cubano	_____	_____
Dominicano	_____	_____
¿Otro grupo?	_____	_____

4. ¿Qué lengua se hablaba en su casa cuando era niño(a)?
   Por favor especifique _____

5. Su fecha de Nacimiento _____
                            (mes)   (dia)   (año)

Cuestionario Acerca de la Etnicidad y el Dolor

Nombre del Paciente _____

Sección A:

(1) ¿Dónde siente usted el dolor?

_____

_____

_____

(2) ¿Qué le causa el dolor?

_____

_____

_____

(3) ¿Cree usted que tiene una clara explicación de su dolor?

_____

_____

(4) ¿Cuánto tiempo hace que tiene usted dolor?

_____

_____

_____

(5) ¿Cuánto tiempo hace que usted viene al médico a causa de su dolor?

_____

_____

_____

Sección B: Para contestar cada pregunta o declaración, ponga un círculo alrededor del número (Ø, 1, 2, 3, 4) de la respuesta más parecida a la suya.

Ø=No es apropiado
1=Estoy fuertemente en desacuerdo
2=Estoy un poco en desacuerdo
3=Estoy de acuerdo hasta cierto punto
4=Estoy muy de acuerdo

(6) Yo tengo todavía muchos de los mismos amigos que tuve de niño(a) y de adolescente.   Ø 1 2 3 4

(7) Vivo en el mismo vecindario o barrio desde mi niñez.   Ø 1 2 3 4

(8) Casi todos mis amigos viven en mi mismo vecindario.   Ø 1 2 3 4

(9) Veo y me reúno con mis hermanos, hermanas o padres con regularidad.   Ø 1 2 3 4

Ø=No es apropiado
1=Estoy fuertemente en desacuerdo
2=Estoy un poco en desacuerdo
3=Estoy de acuerdo hasta cierto punto
4=Estoy muy de acuerdo

(1Ø) Todavía me identifico con las tradiciones
culturales de mi niñez y estas tradiciones
siguen siendo parte de mi vida hoy en día.   Ø 1 2 3 4

(11) Frecuentemente le hablo a otros acerca
de mi dolor.   Ø 1 2 3 4

(12) Me ayuda hablar de mi dolor.   Ø 1 2 3 4

(13) Me emociono cuando describo mi dolor a
los médicos u otras personas.   Ø 1 2 3 4

(14) Cuando el dolor es fuerte, a veces
suspiro y gimo.   Ø 1 2 3 4

(15) No puedo ocultar que tengo dolor.   Ø 1 2 3 4

(16) El dolor no me deja hacer el mismo
trabajo que hacía antes.   Ø 1 2 3 4

(17) Tan pronto como empecé a sentir dolor
dejé de trabajar y me quedé en casa.   Ø 1 2 3 4

(18) Aunque tuve que cambiar mis actividades
debido al dolor, he podido encontrar
otras actividades y trabajo que me manti-
enen activo(a) y ocupado(a).   Ø 1 2 3 4

(19) El dolor hace que me preocupe por lo
que pueda estar mal conmigo.   Ø 1 2 3 4

(2Ø) Pienso mucho en mi dolor.   Ø 1 2 3 4

(21) Mi mayor preocupación es que pueda
tener cáncer u otra enfermedad grave.   Ø 1 2 3 4

(22) Yo pienso mucho en qué habré hecho
para merecer este dolor.   Ø 1 2 3 4

(23) Cuando se descubra la verdadera causa
de mi dolor, no me preocuparé tanto
aunque siga teniendo dolor.   Ø 1 2 3 4

(24) Cuando tengo mucho dolor me siento
muy tenso(a).   Ø 1 2 3 4

(25) Cuando tengo dolor me siento enojado(a). Ø 1 2 3 4

(26) Me siento atemorizado(a) cuando tengo
dolor.   Ø 1 2 3 4

(27) Me siento deprimido(a) cuando tengo
dolor.   Ø 1 2 3 4

(28) Estoy decidido(a) a vencer este dolor.   Ø 1 2 3 4

(29) Jamás tendré una vida feliz o completa
mientras sufra este dolor.   Ø 1 2 3 4

Ø=No es apropiado
1=Estoy fuertemente en desacuerdo
2=Estoy un poco en desacuerdo
3=Estoy de acuerdo hasta cierto punto
4=Estoy muy de acuerdo

(30) Cuando me empezó el dolor fui al médico
inmediatamente.   Ø 1 2 3 4

(31) Yo no creo en tomar medicinas para el
dolor.   Ø 1 2 3 4

(32) Si un médico me dice que una medicina
me va a ayudar yo la tomo exactamente
como me la manda tomar.   Ø 1 2 3 4

(33) Yo he visitado a un quiropráctico.   Ø 1 2 3 4

(34) Si un doctor me da una medicina u
alguna otra indicación y no siento alivio
después de unos días, dejo de tomar la
medicina o no sigo con el tratamiento.   Ø 1 2 3 4

(35) Le he preguntado a mis familiares o
amigos sobre tratamientos para el dolor
y he probado los remedios que me han
sugerido.   Ø 1 2 3 4

(36) He acudido a mi familia y a mis amigos
por ayuda desde que tengo este dolor.   Ø 1 2 3 4

(37) Mi familia y mis amigos me han apoyado
durante los momentos en que he tenido
problemas serios a causa de mi dolor.   Ø 1 2 3 4

Sección C.

(38) Se considera usted   (a) saludable
                                 (b) enfermizo(a)
                                 (c) incapacitado(a)
                                 (d) otro _____
                                     (por favor especifique)

Sección D. Por favor indique si usted cree que las siguientes
           declaraciones son verdaderas o falsas

(39) Las desgracias son el resultado de los
errores que las personas han cometido.   V   F

(40) Desafortunadamente, el valor de una
persona muchas veces no se reconoce a
pesar de sus grandes esfuerzos.   V   F

(41) Muchas de las cosas tristes en la vida
humana se deben en parte a la mala suerte.   V   F

(42) Decidirme a tomar un curso de acción claro
     y definido ha sido mejor para mí que confiar
     en el destino.   V   F

(43) Yo he observado que lo que va a pasar, pasa
     y que yo no tengo control sobre las cosas
     que me pasan.   V   F

(44) Tener éxito en casi todo depende de
     esforzarse en el trabajo. La suerte tiene
     poco o nada que ver con el éxito.   V   F

(45) Cuando yo hago planes estoy casi seguro (a)
     de que saldrán bien.   V   F

(46) Muchas veces siento que no tengo mucho
     control sobre las cosas que me pasan.   V   F

(47) Muchas veces siento que no tengo suficiente
     control sobre la dirección que mi vida
     está tomando.   V   F

(48) Yo creo que tengo control sobre mi dolor y
     que no es el dolor el que determina mi vida.   V   F

APPENDIX E
PAIN CONTROL CENTER QUESTIONNAIRE

1. Patient name: _____

2. Date of birth: _____ 3. Place of birth: _____

4. Male _____ or Female _____

5. Marital Status: _____ 6. Religion _____

7. Are you involved in a workers' compensation case?
   yes _____ no _____

8. When did the pain start?

9. How did it start? _____ accident at home?
   _____ accident at work?
   _____ at work but not an accident?
   _____ after an operation or other physical problem?
   _____ secondary to surgery?
   _____ no apparent cause?

10. Where is your pain located? _____

11. Is the pain: _____ rarely present
    _____ only occurs under certain circumstances
    _____ frequently present
    _____ always present

12. On a scale of 0–10 rate your pain, where 0 MEANS NO PAIN and
    10 MEANS THE WORST PAIN IMAGINABLE
    1. At its worst _____
    2. Usually   _____
    3. At its least _____

13. What medication are you currently using (please list the name
    of each medication)? _____
    _____
    _____

14. Please list any previous surgeries you have had for your pain
    problem. _____
    _____
    _____

15. Please list treatments/therapies for pain, other than
    surgery. _____
    _____
    _____

175

16. Please list any surgeries you have had for problems other than your pain and any other current medical problems which you have. _____

_____

_____

17. Have you been seen by a psychologist or psychiatrist? yes _____ no _____

18. Do you consider yourself to be: (Please circle the correct item)
    a. healthy
    b. unhealthy/disabled
    c. other (please specify) _____

19. Education: Circle the number which indicates the highest level of school completed.

1 2 3 4 5 6 7 8   Grade school
1 2 3 4   High school
1 2 3 4   College
1 2 3 4   Post graduate

20. What is your occupation? _____

21. Are you presently working: _____ full time
                                _____ part time
                                _____ employed but not working since _____
                                unemployed since _____

22. If unemployed, would you like to return to work? _____

23. If yes, doing what work? _____

_____

24. Are you presently suing anyone because of your pain problem? yes _____ no _____

25. What is your yearly income: _____ 7,000 or under
                                _____ 8,000–17,999
                                _____ 18,000–27,999
                                _____ 28,000–37,999
                                _____ 38,000 or over

26. Do you smoke? yes _____ no _____

27. Do you take alcohol? yes _____ no _____

28. Have you lost or gained weight within the past year? yes _____ no _____
    If so, how much: gained _____ lost _____

29. Has your desire for social activities: (please circle one)
    a. remained the same as before the pain
    b. become somewhat less than before the pain
    c. become much less than before the pain
    d. completely disappeared

30. How has your pain effected your ability for social
    activities? (please circle one)
    a. it remains the same as before the pain
    b. it is somewhat less than before the pain
    c. it is much less than before the pain
    d. I am no longer able to engage in social activities
31. What hobbies or recreational activities give you enjoyment?

_____

_____

32. Did you do these activities before your pain started?
    yes _____ no _____
33. Do you enjoy them as much as before your pain?
    yes _____ no _____
34. Do you live: (circle as many as apply)
    a. alone
    b. with spouse
    c. with children
    d. with other relatives
    e. with friends
35. Do you have children? yes _____ no _____
    If so, how many? _____
36. Which of the following are bothering you now? (circle as many
    as apply)
    a. change in job
    b. financial difficulty
    c. marital concerns
    d. family concerns
    e. death of significant other
    f. anything else _____

TABLE OF LEVEL OF INTERFERENCE (TLI)

When you have pain, which of the following activities does your pain affect? Please mark an "X" in the box which best describes to what extent these activities become difficult. If pain is not a problem for you, check here ☐.

	1	2	3	4	0
Activity	Never Difficult	Sometimes Difficult	Fre-quently Difficult	Always Difficult	Not Appli-cable
sleep					
eating					
sports					
schoolwork					
job					
social activities					
household chores					
driving					
walking					
sex					
others (please specify)					

Comments: _____
_____
_____
_____
_____
_____
_____
_____
_____
_____
_____
_____
_____
_____

APPENDIX F

Table F.1. Inter-Ethnic-Group Variation in the MPQ Sensory and Affective Categories

	Anglo American	Latino	Italian	French Canadian	Irish	Polish	F-Ratio	p
SENSORY (MPQ-PRIS)								
Mean	17.8	21.3	19.2	16.9	18.5	16.8	2.34	.04*
SD	7.0	6.3	8.0	7.2	8.0	7.4		
AFFECTIVE (MPQ-PRIA)								
Mean	3.5	6.7	4.1	3.2	3.5	3.3	5.44	.01**
SD	3.9	4.3	3.8	3.6	3.9	3.0		

SD = Standard Deviation

*$p < .05$

**$p < .01$

Table F.2. Multiple Regression Analysis on Pain Intensity (MPQ-PRIT) in the New England Population

VARIABLE	B	+/−	SE B	T	p
Anglo American	−18.23	+/−	5.16	−3.53	.000**
Italian	−3.65	+/−	4.24	−0.86	.390
Fr. Canadian	−7.55	+/−	3.86	−1.95	.052*
Irish	−6.57	+/−	3.90	−1.69	.093
Polish	-30.43	+/−	14.40	−2.11	.036*
Internal LOC	−8.99	+/−	2.88	−3.11	.002**
Age	−.03	+/−	.09	−.33	.074
Polish/LOC	16.79	+/−	15.16	1.11	.270
American/LOC	24.77	+/−	6.67	3.71	.000**
(Constant)	44.70	+/−	4.68	9.54	.000**

R-square = .2205

*$p < .05$

**$p < .01$

(Latino group was the ethnic constant)

Table F.3. Multiple Regressions on Pain Responses in the New England Study Population

Multiple Regression on Work Stoppage[a]

INDEPENDENT VARIABLES	B	+/-	SE B	T	p
Latino	1.36	+/-	.75	1.80	.07
Polish	1.39	+/-	.90	1.53	.13
Italian	1.46	+/-	.72	2.03	.05*
Irish	.86	+/-	.66	1.31	.19
Fr. Canadian	1.45	+/-	.68	2.13	.04*
Workers' Comp.	.96	+/-	.42	2.26	.03*
Education	-.14	+/-	.68	-2.06	.04*
Gender	-.98	+/-	.42	-2.31	.02*
Age	-.22	+/-	.15	-1.45	.15
External LOC	.69	+/-	.40	1.68	.10
Constant	7.22	+/-	-1.53	4.91	.00**

$F = 3.97$, Sig. $= .00**$, R-square $= .28$

Multiple Regression on Pain = Unhappy Life[a]

INDEPENDENT VARIABLES	B	+/-	SE B	T	p
Latino	1.43	+/-	.39	13.26	.00**
Polish	-.35	+/-	.50	.49	.49
Italian	1.01	+/-	.39	6.70	.01**
Irish	-.29	+/-	.36	.64	.94
Fr. Canadian	.68	+/-	.36	3.64	.06
External LOC	.69	+/-	.22	9.69	.00**
Education	-.18	+/-	.24	.24	.62
Constant	1.02	+/-	.61	2.435	.13

$F = 7.27$, Sig. $= .00**$, R-square $= .31$

Multiple Regression on Expressiveness[a]

INDEPENDENT VARIABLES	B	+/-	SE B	T	p
Latino	4.36	+/-	1.15	3.78	.00**
Polish	.86	+/-	1.49	.59	.16
Italian	3.20	+/-	1.11	2.87	.01**
Irish	1.98	+/-	1.03	1.97	.06
Fr. Canadian	1.89	+/-	1.05	1.79	.08
Income 1[c]	1.27	+/-	.89	1.42	.16
Income 2[d]	1.16	+/-	.87	1.35	.18
Income 3[e]	.48	+/-	.94	.52	.61
External LOC	.94	+/-	.66	1.43	.15
Constant	8.22	+/-	1.33	6.11	.00**

Multiple Regression on Anger[b]

INDEPENDENT VARIABLES	B	+/-	SE B	T	p
Anglo American	-.84	+/-	.44	-.19	.85
Italian	.42	+/-	.41	1.02	.31
Fr. Canadian	.25	+/-	.39	.63	.53
Irish	.40	+/-	.43	1.02	.31
Latino	1.01	+/-	.43	2.37	.02*
External LOC	.72	+/-	.20	3.54	.00**
Constant	1.05	+/-	.42	3.66	.00**

$F = 4.96$, Sig. $= .00**$, R-square $= .20$

$F = 3.05$, Sig. $= .00**$, R-square $= .19$
[c]Income Level 1 = 0–$7000 annual
[d]Income Level 2 = $7001–18,000
[e]Income Level 3 = $18,001–28,000
Income Constant was Category 4—$28,000+

(Continued on next page)

Table F.3. (*Cont'd.*)

Multiple Regression on Tension[b]				
INDEPENDENT VARIABLES	B	+/-	SE B	T	p
---	---	---	---	---	---
Anglo American	.20	+/-	.41	.98	.87
Italian	.29	+/-	.29	.99	.38
Fr. Canadian	.21	+/-	.28	.35	.62
Irish	.28	+/-	.32	.34	.45
Latino	1.29	+/-	.31	.37	.00**
Pain Duration	-.20	+/-	.14	.27	.87
Constant	1.42	+/-	.18	6.22	.00**

$F = 3.03$, Sig. = .01**, R-square = .10

Multiple Regression on Worry[b]				
INDEPENDENT VARIABLES	B	+/-	SE B	T	p
---	---	---	---	---	---
Anglo American	-.23	+/-	1.02	-.23	.82
Italian	.94	+/-	.97	.97	.33
Fr. Canadian	.13	+/-	.91	.14	.89
Irish	-.59	+/-	.90	-.65	.95
Latino	2.31	+/-	.99	2.31	.02*
Education	-.59	+/-	.78	-.65	.52
External LOC	1.57	+/-	.48	3.26	.00**
Constant	4.33	+/-	1.41	3.10	.00**

$F = 4.97$, Sig. = .00**, R-square = .23

*p < .05, **p < .01
[a] Anglo American group was the Ethnic Constant
[b] Polish group was the ethnic constant

Table F.4. Multiple Regressions on Care and Treatment Actions
in the New England Study Population

		Multiple Regression Analysis on Immediately Seeks Care of M.D.			
INDEPENDENT VARIABLES	B	+/−	SE B	T	p
External LOC	.30	+/−	.16	1.50	.14
Pain Duration	.51	+/−	.32	.32	.75
Workers' Comp	.66	+/−	.20	3.16	.00*
Constant	2.54	+/−	.32	7.94	.00*

$F = 4.64$ Sig. .004*
R-square = .12

		Multiple Regression on Asking and Using Treatment Advice[a]			
INDEPENDENT VARIABLES	B	+/−	SE B	T	p
Latino	1.29	+/−	.34	3.83	.00*
Polish	.19	+/−	.44	.42	.87
Italian	.29	+/−	.34	−.87	.38
Irish	.23	+/−	.31	.76	.45
Fr. Canadian	.15	+/−	.31	.50	.62
Pain Duration	−.23	+/−	.15	.16	.87
Constant	1.43	+/−	.23	5.85	.00*

$F = 3.03$ Sig. .01*
R-square = .10
*$p < .01$
[a]Anglo American group was the Ethnic Constant

Table F.5. New England Latino and Native Puerto Rican Back-Pain Population
Regression on Pain Intensity (MPQ-PRIT)

INDEPENDENT VARIABLES	B	+/−	SE B	T	p
Puerto Ricans	.27	+/−	.13	2.20	.03*
Internal LOC	−4.92	+/−	3.26	−1.51	.14
Age	−.31	+/−	.15	−2.12	.04*
Education	−.59	+/−	.45	−1.32	.19
Male	.76	+/−	3.48	.22	.83
Duration	.03	+/−	.02	1.52	.00**

$F = 2.32$ Sig. .04**
R-square = .194
*$p < .05$
**$p < .01$

Table F.6. New England Latino and Native Puerto Rican Back-Pain
Population Regression on Anger

INDEPENDENT VARIABLES	B	+/–	SE B	T	p
Puerto Ricans	−.03	+/–	.01	−3.00	.01**
Internal LOC	−.05	+/–	.29	− .16	.87
Age	−.03	+/–	.01	−2.15	.04*
Education	.04	+/–	.04	1.07	.29
Male	.85	+/–	.31	2.72	.01**
Duration	.00	+/–	.01	2.90	.01**

$F = 5.90$ Sig. .00**
R-square = .379
*$p < .05$
**$p < .01$

Table F.7. Multiple Regression on Pain Intensity in the Low-Back-Pain
Population of Anglo Americans and Native Puerto Ricans

VARIABLES	B	+/–	SE B	T	p
Puerto Ricans	.43	+/–	.12	3.51	.00**
LOC	.04	+/–	3.44	.01	.99
Educaiton	−.47	+/–	.53	−90	.37
Age	−.42	+/–	.15	−2.66	.01**
Duration	.04	+/–	.02	2.21	.03*
Male	2.78	+/–	3.72	.74	.45

$F = 5.22$ Sig. $< .00$*
R-square = .416
*$p < .05$
**$p < .01$

GLOSSARY

Afferent nerve fibers: The human body has afferent nerve fibers which conduct nerve impulses from the periphery and internal organs to the central nervous system (the spinal cord and brain), or from lower to higher levels in the sensory projection systems in the spinal cord and brain (Melzack and Wall 1983:405). Because it is important that responses which protect the individual occur before irreversible tissue damage takes place, pain can be felt "following stimuli that are just below levels that cause immediate tissue damage . . . [thus] afferent units that signal tissue injury and inflammation also signal levels of stimulation that only threaten damage" (19).

Causalgia: Reflex sympathetic dystrophy, of which causalgia is one subtype, can occur with an initial injury to nerve, bone, or other soft tissue of an extremity and involves sweating, vasomotor abnormalities, and atrophy as well as severe burning extremity pain which continues after apparent healing has occurred (Berkow 1987:1348). (See *reflex sympathetic dystrophy* definition below for further details.)

Cerebral cortex: The cerebral cortex involves the layers of nerve cells at the outer part of the brain (Melzack and Wall 1988:297).

Dorsal horns: The first six layers of cells in the center of the spinal cord where peripheral nerves enter the spinal cord (Melzack and Wall 1983).

Efferent nerve fibers: Neurons that conduct nerve impulses away from the central nervous system (to muscles or glands) or from higher to lower areas in the nervous system (Melzack and Wall 1988:297).

Hypothalamus: "A portion of the diencephalon of the brain forming the floor and part of the lateral wall of the third ventricle. It activates, controls and integrates the peripheral autonomic nervous system, the endocrine processes, and many somatic functions, such as body temperature, sleep and appetite" (Glanze 1986:560).

Myelin: "A fatty substance surrounding nerve fibers, thereby forming an insulating sheath" (Melzack and Wall 1988:298).

Myelogram: "An x-ray film taken after the injection of a radiopaque medium into the subarachnoid space to demonstrate any distortions of the spinal cord, spinal nerve roots, and the subarachnoid space" (Glanze 1986:743).

Neospinothalmic tract: A long running tract composed of long nerve fibers that connect to the thalamus and to a third relay of fibers that project to the sensory area of the cortex. Information from this pathway arrives rapidly and permits perception of the site, intensity, and duration of noxious stimuli (Chapman 1984:1262–1264).

Neuralgia: "Pain in the distribution of a nerve or nerves" (Melzack and Wall 1988:298).

Neuritis: "The inflammation of a nerve or nerves" (Melzack and Wall 1988:298).

Neuropathy: "A disturbance of function or pathological changes in a nerve" (Melzack and Wall 1988:298).

Neurotransmitters: Chemicals that act at the synapses between neurons; they are responsible for the transmission of nerve impulses across the synaptic junctions and may be excitatory or inhibitory (Saxon 1991:13).

Nociceptors: Receptors that are preferentially sensitive to noxious stimuli or to stimuli which would become noxious if prolonged (Melzack and Wall 1988:298).

Paleospinothalamic tract: A tract composed of long and short fibers that project to various parts of the brain, including the thalamus, reticular formation and the midbrain. This "pathway appears to carry information that produces motivational and emotional dimensions of the pain experience . . . and makes possible the perception of burning, aching, dull and poorly localized pain sensation" (Chapman 1984:1262).

Reflex sympathetic dystrophy: Reflex sympathetic dystrophy can occur with an initial injury to nerve, bone, or other soft tissue of an extremity. It involves autonomic changes (i.e., sweating or vasomotor abnormalities), and/or dystrophic changes (i.e., atrophy of the skin, bone, or joint) and severe, burning pain in the extremity which often continues after the apparent healing of the bone, nerve, or soft tissue (Berkow 1987:1348).

Reticular formation: "A small thick cluster of neurons nestled within the brain stem that controls breathing, the heart beat, the blood pressure, the level of consciousness, and other vital functions of the body. The reticular formation constantly monitors the state of the body through the connections with the sensory and the motor tracks. Certain nerve cells in the formation regulate the flow of hydrochloric acid in the stomach; other cells regulate swallowing, tongue movements and movements of face and eyes" (Glanze 1986:986).

Reticulospinal fibers: The fibers of the reticular formation, some of which project back down to the spinal cord, and others of which extend directly or indirectly to virtually all the areas of the cerebrum (Melzack and Wall 1988:124).

Substantia gelatinosa: The first two layers of cells of the dorsal horns where the A-delta and C nerve fibers enter the spinal cord and connect with the central transmission nerve fibers that project to the brainstem (Melzack and Wall 1983).

Thalamus: The thalamus is "one of the major relay stations of the central nervous system, lying at the top of the brainstem and between the cerebral hemispheres. It relays information projected by the sensory systems to the [cerebral] cortex [the layers of nerve cells at the outer part of the brain] and by the cortex to motor systems or to other brain areas" (Melzack and Wall 1983:409).

Transcutaneous Electrical Nerve Stimulator (TENS unit): "A method of pain control by the application of electric impulses to the nerve endings. This is done through electrodes that are placed on the skin and attached to a stimulator by flexible wires. The electric impulses generated are similar to those of the body, but different enough to block transmission of pain signals to the brain. TENS is noninvasive and nonaddictive, with no side effects" (Glanze 1986:1144).

REFERENCES

Afflek, G., Tennen, H., Pfeiffer, C., and Fifield, J. 1987. Appraisals of Control and Predictability in Adapting to Chronic Diseases. *Journal of Personality and Social Psychology* 54:273–279.

Ahearn, F. Jr. 1979. Puerto Ricans and Mental Health: Some Socio-Cultural Considerations. *The Urban and Social Change Review* 12(2):4–9.

Armelagos, G. J., Goodman, A., and Jacobs, K. 1978. The Ecological Perspective in Disease. In *Health and the Human Condition*, M. Logan and E. Hunt (Eds.), pp. 71–83. North Scituate, MA: Duxbury.

Armelagos, G. J., Leatherman, T., Ryan, M., and Sibley, L. 1992. Biocultural Synthesis in Medical Anthropology. *Medical Anthropology* 14:35–52.

Angel, R., and Guarnaccia, P. 1989. Mind, Body and Culture: Somatization Among Hispanics. *Social Science and Medicine* 28(12):1229–1238.

Aronoff, G. M. 1985. *Evaluation and Treatment of Chronic Pain*. Baltimore: Urban and Schwarzenberg.

Bandura, A. 1977. *Social Learning Theory*. Englewood Cliffs, NJ: Prentice-Hall.

Bastida, E. 1979. Family Integration and Adjustment to Aging Among Hispanic American Elderly. Doctoral Dissertation, University of Kansas. Ann Arbor: University Micro-Films.

Bates, M. S. 1987. Ethnicity and Pain, a Biocultural Model. *Social Science and Medicine* 24:47–50.

Bates, M. S. 1990. A Critical Perspective on Coronary Artery Disease and Coronary Bypass Surgery. *Social Science and Medicine* 30(2):249–260.

Bates, M. S., and Edwards, W. T. 1992. Ethnic Variations in the Chronic Pain Experience. *Ethnicity and Disease* 2(1):63–83.

Bates, M. S., Edwards, W. T., and Anderson, K. 1993. Ethnocultural Influences on Chronic Pain Perception. *Pain* 52:101–112.

Bates, M. S., and Rankin-Hill, L. 1994. Culture, Control and Chronic Pain. *Social Science and Medicine* 39(5):629–645.

Bates, M. S., Rankin-Hill, L., Sanchez-Ayendez, M., and Mendez Bryan, R. 1994. A Cross-Cultural Comparison of Adaptation to Chronic Pain Among Anglo-Americans and Native Puerto Ricans. *Medical Anthropology* 16:1–33.

Bellah, R., et al. 1985. *Habits of the Heart: Individualism and Commitment in American Life*. Berkeley: University of California Press.

Berkow, R. (Ed.). 1987. The Merck Manual. Rahway, NJ: Merck, Sharpe and Dohme Research Laboratories.

Berkowitz, E., and Berkowitz, M. 1989. Incentives for Reducing the Costs of Disability. In *Care and Costs Current Issues in Health Policy*, K. McLennan and J. Meyer (Eds.), pp. 203–226. Boulder: Westview.

Bonica, J. 1953. *The Management of Pain*. Philadelphia: Lea and Febiger.

———. 1985. Introduction. In *Evaluation and Treatment of Chronic Pain*, G. M. Aronoff (Ed.), pp. xxxi–xliv. Baltimore: Urban and Schwarzenberg.

Bonica J., and Chapman, R. 1986. Biology, Pathophysiology and Therapy of Chronic Pain. In *American Handbook of Psychiatry*, (2nd ed., vol. 8), S. Arieti (Ed.), pp. 721–722, New York: Basic.

Brennan, A. F., Barrett, C. L., Garretson, H. D. 1987. The Prediction of Chronic Pain Outcome by Psychological Variables. *International Journal of Psychiatry in Medicine* 16:373–387.

Buckelew, S.P., Shutty, M.S. Jr., Hewett, J., Landon, T., Morrow, K., Frank, R. G. 1990. Health Locus of Control, Gender Differences and Adjustment to Persistent Pain. *Pain* 42(3):287–294.

Buitrago, C. 1966. La investigacion social y el problem de los investigadores puertorriquenos en las ciencias sociales y disciplinas relacionadas en P. R. *Revista de Ciencias Sociales 9* (1):93–103.

———. 1970. Estructura social y orientaciones valorativas en Esperanza, Puerto Rico y el Mediterraneo. Editorial Edil, San Juan, Puerto Rico.

Buitrago-Ortiz, C., Pacheco-Maldonado, A., and Garriga-Pico, J. 1981. La cultura como contexto, proceso, producto y proyecto de la accion humna. *Revista de Ciencias Sociales* 23(1–2):253–264.

Bureau of the Census. 1980. Census of the Population Vol. 1, Characteristics of the Population, Chapter C, General Social and Economic Characteristics, Part 23, Massachusetts. Washington, D.C.: U.S. Department of Commerce.

Burgos, N., and Diaz Perez, Y. 1986. An Exploration of Human Sexuality in the Puerto Rican Culture. *Journal of Social Work and Human Sexuality* 4:135–150.

Buss, A., and Portnoy, N. 1967. Pain Tolerance and Group Identification. *Journal of Personality and Social Psychology* 6:106–108.

Canino, G., Rubio-Stipec, M., Shrout, P., Bravo, M., Stolberg, R., Bird, H. 1987. Sex Differences and Depression In Puerto Rico. *Psychology of Women Quarterly* 11:443–459.

Canino, G., Braveo, M., Rubio-Stipec, M., and Woodbury, M. 1990. The Impact of Disaster on Mental Health: Prospective and Retrospective Analyses. *International Journal Of Mental Health* 19:51–69.

Canino, I. A., and Canino, G. J. 1980. Impact of Stress on the Puerto Rican Family. *American Journal of Orthopsychiatry* 50(3):535–541.

————. 1993. Psychiatric Care of Puerto Ricans. In *Culture, Ethnicity and Mental Illness*, A. C. Gaw (Ed.), pp. 467–499. Washington, D.C.: American Psychiatric Press.

Chapman, C. R. 1984. New Directions in the Understanding and Management of Pain. *Social Science and Medicine* 19:1261–1277.

Coreil, J., and Marshall, P. A. 1982. Locus of Illness Control: A Cross-Cultural Study. *Human Organizations* 41:131–138.

Craig, K. D. 1983. A Social Learning Perspective on Pain Experience. In M. Rosenbaum, Cyril, M. Franks, Yoram Jaffe (eds.) *Perspectives on Behavior Therapy in the Eighties*, pp. 311-327. New York: Springer.

Craig, K. D., and Neidermayer, H. 1974. Autonomic Correlates of Pain Thresholds Influenced by Social Modeling. *Journal of Personality and Social Psychology* 29:246–252.

Departamento de Salud. 1988. *Informe Anual de Estadisticas Vitales, Division de Estadisticas*. San Juan, Puerto Rico: Departamento de Salud.

————. 1989, February. *Ofinica de Planificacion, Evaluacion e Informes—Boletin Informativo* (Serie D-6:2). Santruce, Puerto Rico: Departamento de Salud.

Departamento de Trabajo. 1989. *Encuesta de Vivienda*. San Juan, Puerto Rico: Departamento de Trabajo.

Diamond, A. W., and Coniam, S. W. 1991. *The Management of Chronic Pain*. Oxford: Oxford University Press.

Dorsel, T. 1989. Chronic Pain Behavior Patterns, a Simple Theoretical Framework for Health Care Providers. *Psychological Reports* 65:783–786.

Duany, J. 1988-89. Cultura y Personalidad en Puerto Rico: para una Psicologia de la Identidad Nacional. *Homines* 12(1–2):180–185.

Duran, R. P. 1983. *Hispanics' Education and Background: Predictors of College Achievement*. New York: College Entrance Exam Boards.

Dworkin, R. H., Richlin, D., Handlin, D., and Brand, L. 1986. Predicting Treatment Response in Depressed and Non-Depressed Chronic Pain Patients. *Pain* 24:343–353.

Edwards, P., O'Neil, G., Zeichner, S., and Kuczmierczyk, A. 1985. Effects of Familial Pain Models on Pain Complaints and Coping Strategies. *Perception and Motor Skills* 61:1053–1054.

Edwards, P., Zeichner, S., Kuczmierczyk, A., and Boczkowski, J. 1985. Familial Pain Models: the Relationship Between Family History of Pain and Current Pain Experiences. *Pain* 21:379–384.

Edwards, W., Habib, F., Burney, R., and Begin, G. 1985. Intravenous Lidocaine in the Management of Various Chronic Pain States. *Regional Anesthesia* 10:1–6.

Elton, D., Burrows, G. D., Stanley, G. V. 1979. Clinical Measurement of Pain. *The Medical Journal of Australia* 24:109–111.

Estes, G., and Zitzow, D. 1980. Heritage Consistency as a Consideration in Counseling Native Americans. Paper presented at the National Indian Education Association Convention, Dallas, Texas, November.

Fields, H., and Basbaum, A. 1989. Endogenous Pain Control Mechanisms. In P. Wall. and R. Melzack (Eds.), *Textbook of Pain*, pp. 206–217. New York: Churchill Livingstone.

Finkler, K. 1991. *Physicians at Work, Patients in Pain.* Boulder: Westview.

Flor, H., and Turk, D. 1989. Psychophysiology of Chronic Pain: Do Chronic Pain Patients Exhibit Symptom-Specific Psychophysiological Responses? *Psychological Bulletin* 105(2):215–259.

Fordyce, W. 1976. *Behavioral Methods for Chronic Pain and Illness.* St. Louis: C. V. Mosby.

Fordyce, W., Roberts, A., and Sternbach, R. 1985. The Behavioral Management of Chronic Pain: A Response to Critics. *Pain* 22:113–125.

Fotopoulos, S. S., Graham, C., and Cook, M. 1979. Psychophysiologic Control of Cancer Pain. In *Advances in Pain Research and Therapy (vol. 3)*, Bonica J. (Ed.), pp. 231–43. New York: Raven.

Fox, E., and Melzack, R. 1976. Comparison of Transcutaneous Electrical Stimulation and Acupuncture in the Treatment of Chronic Pain. In *Advances in Pain Research and Therapy (vol. 1)*, J. Bonica and D. Albe-Fessard (Eds.), pp. 797–801. New York: Raven.

Garfield, E. 1980. Most Cited Articles of the 1960s. Preclinical Basic Research. *Current Contents* 23(5):5–13.

Garza, R. T., and Widlak, F. W. 1977. The Validity of Locus of Control Dimensions for Chicano Populations. *Journal of Personality Assessment* 41:635–643.

Gaston-Johansson, F., Johansson, G., Felldin, R., and Sanne, H. 1985. A Comparative Study of Pain Description, Emotional Discomfort and Health Perception in Patients with Chronic Pain Syndrome and Rheumatoid Arthritis. *Scandinavian Journal of Rehabilitative Medicine* 17:109–119.

Gentry. W., Shows, W., and Thomas, M. 1974. Chronic Low-Back Pain: A Psychological Profile. *Psychosomatics* 15:174–177.

Ghali, S. B. 1977, October. Culture Sensitivity and the Puerto Rican Client. *Social Casework* 58:459–474.

———. 1982, January. Understanding Puerto Rican Traditions. *Social Work* 27:98–102.

Gilbert, M. 1989. Cultural Relevance in the Delivery of Human Services. In *Negotiating Ethnicity: The Impact of Anthropological Theory and Practice*, S.

Keefe (Ed.), pp. 39–48. Washington, D.C.: National Association for the Practice of Anthropology.

Glanze, W. D. (Ed.) 1986. *Mosby's Medical and Nursing Dictionary* (2nd ed.). St. Louis: C. V. Mosby.

Good, B. J., and Good, M. D. 1980. The Meaning of Symptoms: A Cultural Hermeneutic Model for Clinical Practice. In *Relevance of Social Science for Medicine*, L. Eisenberg, and A. Kleinman (Eds.), pp. 165–196. Dordrecht, Holland: Reidel.

Good, M. J. 1992. Work as a Haven from Pain. In *Pain as Human Experience: An Anthropological Perspective*, Good, M. J., Brodwin, P., Good, B., and Kleinman, A., pp. 49–76. Berkeley: University of California Press.

Good, M. J., Brodwin, P., Good, B., and Kleinman, A. 1992. *Pain as Human Experience: An Anthropological Perspective*. Berkeley: University of California Press.

Gracely, R. H. 1984. Subjective Quantification of Pain Perception. In: *Pain Measurement in Man*, B. Bromm (Ed.), pp. 371–387. Amsterdam: Elsevier Science Publishers.

Greenwald, H. P. 1991. Interethnic Differences in Pain Perception. *Pain* 44:157–163.

Guagnano, G., Acredolo, C., Hawkes, G. Ellyson, S., and White, N. 1986. Locus of Control: Demographic Factors and Their Interactions. *Journal of Social Behavior and Personality* 1(3):365–380.

Guarnaccia, P. J. 1993. *Ataques De Nervios* in Puerto Rico: Culture-Bound Syndrome or Popular Illness? *Medical Anthropology* 15(2):157–170.

Harwood, A. 1977. *Rx: Spiritist as Needed. A Study of a Puerto Rican Community Mental Health Resource*. New York: John Wiley and Sons.

Herman, E. W. 1990. Group Experience as Healing Process. In *Chronic Pain* (vol. 2), T. W. Miller (Ed.), pp. 459–497. Madison: International Universities Press.

Holzman, A. D., and Turk, D. C. (Eds.). 1986. *Pain Management*. Oxford: Pergamon.

House, J., Landis, K., and Umberson, D. 1990. Social Relationships and Health. In *The Sociology of Health and Illness Critical Perspectives*, P. Conrad and R. Kern (Eds.), pp. 85–94. New York: St. Martin's.

Jacobson, D. 1987. The Cultural Context of Social Support and Support Networks. *Medical Anthropology Quarterly* 1(1):42–67.

Jensen, M. P., and Karoly, P. 1991. Pain-Specific Beliefs, Perceived Symptom Severity, and Adjustment to Chronic Pain. *Clinical Journal of Pain* 8:123–130.

Jordan, B. 1993. *Birth in Four Cultures* (4th ed.). Prospect Heights, IL: Waveland.

Keefe, R., and Gill, K. 1985. Recent Advances in the Behavioral Assessment and Treatment of Chronic Pain. *Annals of Behavioral Medicine* 7:11–16.

Kist-Kline, G., and Lipnickey, S. 1989. Health Locus of Control: Implications for the Health Professional. *Health Values* 13(55):38–47.

Kleinman, A. 1980. *Patients and Healers in the Context of Culture.* Berkeley: University of California Press.

———. 1986. *Social Origins of Distress and Disease: Depression, Neurasthenia and Pain in Modern China.* New Haven: Yale University Press.

———. 1988. *The Illness Narratives.* New York: Basic.

Kleinman, A., Eisenberg, L., and Good, B. 1978. Clinical Lessons from Anthropologic and Cross-Cultural Research. *Annals of Internal Medicine* 88:251–258.

Knox, V., Shum, K., and McLaughlin, D. 1977. Response to Cold Pressor Pain and to Acupuncture Analgesia in Oriental and Occidental Subjects. *Pain* 4:49–57.

Kores, R., Murphy, W. D., Rosenthal, T. L., Elias, D. B., North, W. C. 1990. Predicting Outcome of Chronic Pain Treatment Via a Modified Self-Efficacy Scale. *Behavioral Research Therapy* 28(2):165–169.

Koss, J. 1980. The Therapist-Spiritist Training Project in Puerto Rico: An Experiment to Relate the Traditional Healing System to the Public Health System. *Social Science and Medicine* 14(B):255–266.

———. 1987. Expectations and Outcomes for Patients Given Mental Health Care or Spiritist Healing in Puerto Rico. *American Journal of Psychiatry* 144(1):56–61.

Koss-Chioino, J. 1992. *Women as Healers, Women as Patients.* Boulder: Westview.

Kotarba, J. 1983. *Chronic Pain, Its Social Dimensions.* Beverly Hills: Sage.

Krause, N., and Stryker, S. 1984. Stress and Well-being: The Buffering Role of Locus of Control Beliefs. *Social Science and Medicine* 18:783–790.

Lahuerta, J., Smith, B., and Martinez-Lage, J. 1982. An Adaptation of The McGill Pain Questionnaire to the Spanish Language. *Schmerz* 3:32–34.

Lauria, A. 1964. Respeto, Relajo, and Interpersonal Relations in Puerto Rico. *Anthropological Quarterly* 37:53–67.

Lawlis, G. F., Achterberg, J., Kenner, L., and Kopetz, K. 1984. Ethnic and Sex Differences in Response to Clinical and Induced Pain in Chronic Spinal Pain Patients. *Spine* 9:751–754.

Lefcourt, H. 1980. Locus of Control and Coping with Life's Events. In *Personality*, E. Staub (Ed.). Englewood Cliffs, NJ: Prentice Hall.

Leiderman, D. 1977. Cross-Cultural Inferences of Physical Pain and Psychological Distress-1. *Nursing Times* 73:521–558.

Leroy, P. L. 1977. *Current Concepts in the Management of Chronic Pain.* Miami: Symposia Specialists.

Linton, S., and Gotestam, K. 1985. Controlling Pain Reports Through Operant Conditioning: A Laboratory Demonstration. *Perceptions and Motor Skills* 60:427–437.

Linton, S. J. 1982. A Critical Review of Behavioral Treatments for Chronic Benign Pain other than Headache. *British Journal of Clinical Psychology* 21:321–330.

Lipton, S. 1990. Introduction. In *Advances in Pain Research and Therapy* (vol. 13). S. Lipton, E. Tunks, and M. Zoppi (Eds.), pp. xxvii–xxxiii. New York: Raven.

Lipton, J. A., and Marbach, J. J. 1984. Ethnicity and the Pain Experience. *Social Science and Medicine* 19:1279–1298.

Lyndsay, P., and Wyckoff, M. 1981. The Depression-Pain Syndrome and Its Response to Antidepressants. *Psychosomatics* 22:571–577.

Maciewicz, R., and Sandrew, B. 1985. Physiology of Pain. In *Evaluation and Treatment of Chronic Pain*, G. Aronoff, (Ed.), pp. 17–31. Baltimore: Urban and Schwarzenberg.

Malec, J., Cayner, J., Harvey, R., and Timming R. 1981. Pain Management: Long-Term Follow-Up of an Inpatient Program. *Archives of Physical Medicine and Rehabilitation* 62:369–372.

Marin, G., and VanOss Marin, B. 1991. *Research with Hispanic Populations*. Newbury Park, CA: Sage.

Marin, G., and Triandis, H. 1985. Allocentrism as an Important Characteristic of the Behavior of Latin Americans and Hispanics. In *Cross-Cultural and National Studies in Social Psychology*, R. Diaz-Guerrero (Ed.), pp. 85–104. Amsterdam: Elsevier Science Publishers.

Marshall, P. 1991. Debate Over Puerto Rico's Political Status. *Editorial Research Reports* (February 8):82–95.

McNeil, T., Sinkora, G., and Levavitt, F. 1986. Psychological Classification of Low Back Pain Patients: A Prognostic Tool. *Spine* 11:95–99.

Mechanic, D. 1972. Social Psychological Factors Affecting the Presentation of Bodily Complaints. *New England Journal of Medicine* 286:1132–1139.

Melzack, R., 1975. The McGill Pain Questionnaire: Major Properties and Scoring Methods. *Pain* 1:277–299.

———. 1984. Measurement of the Dimensions of Pain Experience. In *Pain Measurement in Man*, B. Bromm (Ed.), pp. 327–347. Amsterdam: Elsevier Science Publishers.

Melzack, R., and Torgenson, W. 1971. On the Language of Pain. *Anesthesiology* 34:50–59.

Melzack, R. and Wall, P. 1965. Pain Mechanisms: A New Theory. *Science* 150:971–979.

———. 1970. Psychophysiology of Pain. *International Anesthesiology of Clinics Quarterly* 8:3–34.

———. 1983, 1988. *The Challenge of Pain*. New York: Penguin.

Melzack, R., Weisz, A., and Sprague, L. 1963. Stratagems for Controlling Pain: Contributions of Auditory Stimulation and Suggestion. *Experience and Neurology* 8:239–243.

Merskey, H. 1979. Pain Terms: A List with Definitions and Notes on Usage, Recommended by the IASP Subcommittee on Taxonomy. *Pain* 6:249–252.

———. 1986. International Association for the Study of Pain, Classifications of Chronic Pain. *Pain* (Supplement 3):S1–S225.

———. 1987. Pain, Personality and Psychosomatic Complaints. In *Handbook of Chronic Pain Management*, G. Burrows, E. Elton, and G. Stanley (Eds.), pp. 137–146. Amsterdam: Elsevier Scientific Press.

Merskey, H. and Magni, G. 1990. Psychological Techniques in the Treatment of Chronic Pain. In *Chronic Pain* (vol. 2), T. W. Miller (Ed.), pp. 367–388. Madison: International Universities Press.

Miller, T. W. (Ed.) 1990. *Chronic Pain* (vol. 2). Madison: International Universities Press.

Mintz, S. 1975. Puerto Rico: An Essay in the Definition of a National Culture. In *The Puerto Rican Experience, Status of Puerto Rico: Selected Background Studies*, United States–Puerto Rico Commission on the Status of Puerto Rico, pp. 339–434. New York: Arno.

Molina, J., Coppo, C., and del Docente, P. 1984. The Argentine Pain Questionnaire. *Pain* (Supplement 2), Abstracts of the Fourth World Congress on Pain.

Morales Carrion, A. 1983. *Puerto Rico: A Political and Cultural History*. New York: W. W. Norton.

Morales, J. 1986. *Puerto Rican Poverty and Migration: We Just Had to Try Elsewhere*. New York: Praeger.

Morris, D. 1991. *The Culture of Pain*. Berkeley: University of California Press.

Mountcastle. V. B. 1974. *Medical Physiology*. St. Louis: C. V. Mosby.

Osterweis, M., Kleinman, A., and Mechanic, D. (Eds.) 1987. *Pain and Disability*. Washington, D.C.: National Academy Press.

Pickens, I., and Ireland, G. 1969. Family Patterns of Medical Care Utilization. *Journal of Chronic Diseases* 22:181–191.

Pilowski, I., and Spence, N. 1976. Illness Behavior Syndromes Associated with Intractable Pain. *Pain* 2:61–71.

Pither, C. E., and Nicholas, M. K. 1991. Psychological Approaches in Chronic Pain Management. *British Medical Bulletin* 47:743–761.

Prieto, E., Hopson, L., Bradley, L., Bryne, M., Geisinger, K., Midax, D. and Marchisello, P. 1980. The Language of Low Back Pain: Factor Structure of the McGill Pain Questionnaire. *Pain* 8:11–20.

Ramirez, R. L. 1973. Rituales Politics en Puerto Rico. *Revista de Ciencias Sociales* 17(3):309–323.

———. 1992. Power, Pleasure and Pain: Puerto Rican Male Discourses. Paper presented at the 91st annual meeting of the American Anthropological Association, San Francisco, December 2–6.

Reid, V., and Bush, J. 1990. Ethnic Factors Influencing Pain Expression: Implication for Clinical Assessment. In *Chronic Pain* (vol. 1), T. Miller (Ed.), pp. 117–145. Madison: International Universities Press.

Reyes, J., and Inclan, J. 1991. *A Study of the Mental Health Treatment of the Puerto Rican Migrant.* M.E.R.T.I. Minority Education Research and Training Institute, Monograph No. 1. New York: The Minority Education, Research and Training Institute at Metropolitan Hospital, Community Mental Health Center, New York City Health and Hospitals Corporation.

Rifkin, J. 1987. *Time Wars: The Primary Conflict in Human History.* New York: Henry Holt.

Robles, R., Alegria, M., Martinez, R., Vera, M., and Munoz, C. 1982. Social Integration and Health Among Puerto Rican Return Migrants. *Puerto Rico Health Sciences Journal* 1:119–125.

Rodriguez, C. E. 1991. *Puerto Ricans Born in the U.S.A.* Boulder: Westview.

Rogler, L., Cortes, D., and Malgady, R. 1991. Acculturation and Mental Health Status Among Hispanics. *American Psychologist* 46:585–597.

Roemer, M. I. 1991. *National Health Systems of the World.* Vol. 1. New York: Oxford University Press.

Rotheram, M. J., and Phinney, J. 1987. Introduction, Definitions and Perspectives in the Study of Children's Ethnic Socialization. In *Children's Ethnic Socialization*, J. Phinney and M. Rotheram (Eds.), pp. 10–28. Newbury Park: Sage.

Rotter, J. B. 1966. Generalized Expectancies for Internal Versus External Control of Reinforcement. New York: American Psychological Association Monographs.

Rubin, L. B. 1976. *Worlds of Pain: Life in the Working-Class Family.* New York: Basic.

Sanchez-Ayendez, M. 1984. Puerto Rican Elderly Women: Aging in an Ethnic Minority Group in the United States. Doctoral Dissertation, University of Massachusetts-Amherst. Ann Arbor: University Micro-Films.

———. 1988. Puerto Rican Elderly Women: The Cultural Dimension of Social Support Networks. *Women and Health* 14(3–4):239–252.

———. 1992. Puerto Rican Elderly Women: Shared Meanings and Informal Supportive Networks. In *Race, Class, and Gender*, M. Andersen and P. Collins (Eds.). Berkeley: Wadsworth.

———. 1993. Informal Carers to the Elderly: A Holistic Perspective. Paper prepared for the World Development Bank, World Development Report, 1993 (presented at the Consultation Meeting on Health of the Elderly, Oslo, Norway, November 1992).

Sargent, C. 1986. Between Death and Shame: Dimensions of Pain in Bariba Culture. *Social Science and Medicine* 19:1299–1304.

———. 1989. *Maternity, Medicine, and Power.* Berkeley: University of California Press.

Saxon, S. V. 1991. *Pain Management Techniques for Older Adults.* Springfield, IL: Charles C. Thomas.

Schensul, J., Nieves, I., and Martinez, M. 1982. The Crisis Event in the Puerto Rican Community: Research and Intervention in the Community/Institution Interface. *Urban Anthropology 11*(1):101–128.

Seda-Bonilla, E. 1964. Interraccion social y personalidad en una communidad de Puerto Rico. Ediciones Ponce de Leon, San Juan, Puerto Rico.

———. 1970. Requiem por una cultura: ensayos sobre la socializacion del Puertorriqueno en su cultura y en ambito del poder neocolonial. Editoral Edil, Rio Piedras, Puerto Rico.

Sheridan, M. S. 1992. *Pain in America.* Tuscaloosa: University of Alabama Press.

Sherif, M., and Sherif, C. W. 1964. *Reference Groups.* New York: Harper and Row.

Shorben, E., and Borland, L. 1954. An Empirical Study of Etiology of Dental Fears. *Journal of Clinical Psychology 10*:171–174.

Spector, R. E. 1985. *Cultural Diversity in Health and Illness.* Norwalk, CT: Appleton-Century-Crofts.

Spence, S. 1991. Case History and Shorter Communication. *Behavioral Research and Therapy 29*(5):503–509.

Stans, L., Goossens, L., Van Houdenhove, B., Adriaensen, H., Verstraeten, D., Vervaeke, M., and Fannes, V. 1989. Evaluation of a Brief Chronic Pain Management Program: Effects and Limitations. *Clinical Journal of Pain* 5:317–322.

Stein, H. 1990. *American Medicine as Culture.* Boulder: Westview.

Stenger, E. M. 1992. Chronic Back Pain: A View from a Psychiatrist's Office. *Clinical Journal of Pain 8*:242–246.

Sternbach, R. A. 1974. *Pain Patients' Traits and Treatments.* New York: Academic Press.

———. 1984. Behavior Therapy. In *The Textbook of Pain*, P. Wall and R. Melzack (Eds.), pp. 800–805. New York: Churchill Livingstone.

Steward, J., Manners, R., Wolf, E., Padilla, E., Mintz, S., and Scheele, R. 1956. *The People of Puerto Rico: A Study in Social Anthropology.* Urbana: University of Illinois Press.

Streltzer, J., and Wade, T. 1981. The Influence of Cultural Group on the Undertreatment of Post-Operative Pain. *Psychosomatic Medicine 43*:392–403.

Swanson, D. 1984. Chronic Pain as a Third Pathological Emotion. *American Journal of Psychiatry 14*:210–214.

Swanson, D., Maruta, T., and Swenson, W. 1979. Results of Behavior Modification in the Treatment of Chronic Pain. *Psychosomatic Medicine 1*:55–61.

Szalay, L., and Diaz-Guerrero, R. 1985. Similarities and Differences Between Subjective Cultures: A Comparison of Latin, Hispanic, and Anglo Americans. In *Cross-Cultural and National Studies in Social Psychology*, R.

Diaz-Guerrero (Ed.), pp. 105–133. Amsterdam: Elsevier Science Publishers.

Talo, S., Hendler, N., and Brodie, J. 1989. Effects of Active and Completed Litigation on Treatment Results: Workers' Compensation Patients Compared with Other Litigation Patients. *Journal of Occupational Medicine* 31(3):265–269.

Tait, R., Chibnall, J., and Richardson, W. 1990. Litigation and Employment Status: Effects on Patients with Chronic Pain. *Pain* 43:37–46.

Tait, R., De Good, D., and Carron, H. 1982. A Comparison of Health Locus of Control Beliefs in Low-Back Patients from the U.S. and New Zealand. *Pain* 14:53–61.

Tienda, M. 1985. The Puerto Rican Worker: Current Labor Market Status and Future Prospects. In *Puerto Ricans in the Mid '80s: An American Challenge*, Alexandria, VA: National Puerto Rican Coalition.

Todd, E. 1985. Pain: Historical Perspectives. In *Evaluation and Treatment of Chronic Pain*, G. M. Aronoff (Ed.), pp. 1–16. Baltimore: Urban and Schwarzenberg.

Tollison, C. D., Kriegel, M. L., Satterthwaite, J. R., Hinnant, D. W., Turner, K. P. 1989. Comprehensive Pain Center Treatment of Low Back Workers' Compensation Injuries. *Orthopedic Review* 18(10):1115–1126.

Tropman, J. E. 1989. *American Values and Social Welfare*. Englewood Cliffs, NJ: Prentice Hall.

Turk, D. C. 1993. Assess the Person, Not Just the Pain. *Pain Clinical Updates* 1(3):1–4.

Turk, D., Flor, H., and Rudy, T. 1987. Pain and Families I: Etiology, Maintenance, and Psychosocial Impact. *Pain* 30:3–27.

Turk, D., and Kerns, R. 1985. *Health, Illness and Families: A Life-Span Perspective.* New York: Wiley-Interscience.

Turk, D., and Meichenbaum, D. 1989. A Cognitive-Behavioral Approach to Pain Management. In *The Textbook of Pain*, P. Wall and R. Melzack (Eds.), pp. 1001–1009. New York: Churchill Livingstone.

Turk, D., Meichenbaum, D., and Genest, M. 1983. *Pain and Behavioral Medicine: A Cognitive-Behavioral Perspective*. New York: Guilford.

Turk, D., Rudy, T., and Salovey, P. 1985. The McGill Pain Questionnaire Reconsidered: Confirming the Factor Structure and Examining Appropriate Uses. *Pain* 21:385–397.

Turner, J., and Clancy, S. 1988. Comparison of Operant Behavioral and Cognitive-Behavioral Group Treatment for Chronic Low Back Pain. *Journal of Consulting and Clinical Psychology* 56:261–266.

Violon, A., and Giurgea, D. 1984. Familial Models for Chronic Pain. *Pain* 18:199–203.

Waitzkin, H. 1993. *The Second Sickness: Contradictions of Capitalist Health Care.* New York: The Free Press.

Wall, P., and Jones, M. 1991. *Defeating Pain: The War Against a Silent Epidemic.* New York: Plenum.

Wall P., and Melzack, R. 1984, 1989. *The Textbook of Pain.* New York: Churchill Livingstone.

Weidman, H. H. 1979. The Transcultural View: Prerequisite to Interethnic (Intercultural) Communication in Medicine. *Social Science and Medicine 13*(B):85–87.

Weisenberg, M. 1977. Pain and Pain Control. *Psychological Bulletin 84*:1008–1044.

Weisenberg, M., Kreindler, L., Schachat, R., and Werboff, J. 1975. Pain: Anxiety and Attitudes in Black, White, and Puerto Rican Patients. *Psychosomatic Medicine 37*:123–135.

Weisman, A. 1990. An Island in Limbo. *New York Times Magazine* (February 18): 29–36.

Westbrook, M. T., Nordholm, L., and McGee, J. 1984. Cultural Differences in Reactions to Patient Behavior: A Comparison of Swedish and Australian Health Professionals. *Social Science and Medicine 19*:939–947.

Wooley, S., and Epps, B. 1975. Pain Tolerance in Chronic Illness Behavior. *Psychosomatic Medicine 37*:98.

Wright, J., Gerschmann, J., Reade, P., and Holwill, B. 1983. Comparison of Socio-Cultural Factors in Patients with Oro-Facial Pain and Dental Phobias. *Journal of Dental Research 62*:670.

Wuthnow, R. 1994. *Sharing the Journey: Support Groups and America's Quest for Community.* New York: The Free Press; Macmillan.

Zayas, L., and Palleja, J. 1988. Puerto Rican Familism: Considerations for Family Therapy. *Family Relations 37*:260–264.

Zborowski, M. 1952. Cultural Components in Responses to Pain. *Journal of Social Issues 8*:16–30.

———. 1969. *People in Pain.* San Francisco: Jossey-Bass.

Zola, I. K. 1966. Culture and Symptoms—An Analysis of Patients Presenting Complaints. *American Sociological Review 31*:615–630.

INDEX

Nociceptors, 8
Norepinephrine, 10
Nutritional counseling, 23, 27

Occupational therapy, 23, 27, 51, 64, 67, 69, 144
Operant conditioning, 18
Operation Bootstrap, 100
Osteoarthritis, 77
Osteoporosis, 118

Pain: acute, 17, 20, 43; altering interpretations of, 19–20; assessment of, 3; attitudes toward, 17, 32; behavior, xvi, xvii, 18, 21, 50, 64, 78, 116, 137; biocultural model of perception, 54–57, 56*fig*; biological aspects of, 21; "career," 59; causalgia, 8; cognitive processes in, xvii, 8, 19–20; cultural influences, 13–18; defining, 7; descriptions of, 31; as diagnostic aid, 17; essential nature of, xv; experimental, 43; function of, xv, xvi, 11; genetic variables in, 14; intensity, 13, 136–137; meanings for, 17, 53–54, 138; memories of, 15; modulation of, 12, 13; overcoming, 32; perception, xvi, 7–13, 138; phantom limb, 8; physiological components of, xvii; preoccupation with, 1; psychological processes in, xvi, xvii, 8; reflex sympathetic dystrophy, 8; sensation, 11–12; social influences, 13–18; sociocultural components of, xvii; subjective nature of, 7, 56; theories of, xvi, 7–23; thresholds, 9, 10; tolerance, 14; transmission, 12; understanding of, 27
Pain, chronic, 38; adaptation to, 2, 26, 32, 59, 135; and age, 44, 45*fig*, 88, 105, 121, 123*tab*; attitudinal responses to, 83, 123–124, 131–132; behavioral responses to, 80, 83, 123, 129, 130*tab*; "career," xvi, xvin, 25; case studies, 2–6, 49–54, 61–65, 67–79; control over, 3; coping strategies, 2, 3, 4, 26, 53, 60, 71–72, 73, 114, 124; defining, 28; degenerative disks, 38; as disability, 17; duration differences, 121–122, 123*tab*; economic costs of, xv; educational differences, 121, 123*tab*, 125*tab*; effect on behavior, 25; effect on sexual relations, 68, 71, 72,

131*tab*; emotional responses to, 83–84, 123, 130–131; and employment, 2, 3, 4; and ethnicity, 15–18, 25–41, 43–49; expressing, 3, 32; gender differences, 125*tab*; governmental concern over, 19; intensity differences, 122, 124*tab*, 127, 136–137; inter-ethnic variations, 80, 81–82*tab*, 83–84, 128–132; intra-ethnic variations, 84–88, 89–91*tab*, 92–94; and locus-of-control, 44, 45*fig*, 47, 48*fig*, 49, 105, 107, 107*tab*, 115; low-back, 38, 38n, 50, 52, 61, 63, 67, 71, 77; measures of intensity, 28; mechanical, 38; in other family members, 14; postsurgical, 38; psychological responses to, 7, 83–84, 123, 130–131; as psychosocial disturbance, 20; role of family in, 14; search for cure, 26; and social activities, 3, 52, 68, 71, 74, 107, 116, 131*tab*; and social relationships, 25; socioeconomic hardship of, 17; and socioeconomic status, 88, 90*tab*, 92; stress of, 17; study conclusions, 135–156; support groups, 148; variations in intensities, 31, 43–57; variations in response to, 59–97
Paleospinothalamic tract, 11
Patient(s): age differences, 121, 123*tab*; attitudes as predictors of adjustment, 83n; biocultural environment of, 136–145; characteristics of, 1–2; diversity among, xvi, 2, 135; educational differences, 121, 123*tab*, 125*tab*; and ethnicity, 45*fig*; gender differences, 125*tab*; pain duration differences, 121–122, 123*tab*; pain intensity differences, 122, 124*tab*, 127; psychosocial environment of, 145–149; resocialization of, 143
Patients in New England, 25–41, 121–134; age groups, 30*tab*, 38, 47, 80, 88, 89*tab*, 181–184*tab*; Anglo American group, 28–29, 30*tab*, 36, 37*fig*, 38, 44, 46, 49, 52–54, 60–65, 81–82*tab*, 83, 86, 87, 88, 89*tab*, 90*tab*, 93*tab*, 181–184*tab*; case studies, 49–54, 61–65, 67–79; characteristics, 27–29, 30*tab*; cognitive styles of, 39–41; comparisons with Puerto Rican patients, 121–134; cultural characteristics of, 36–38; description of health status, 82*tab*, 83, 87; diagnoses, 30*tab*, 46, 50; duration of chronic pain, 30*tab*, 38;